General Principles of Surgery

Handbooks in General Surgery

T0235489

Kirby I. Bland • Michael G. Sarr
Markus W. Büchler • Attila Csendes
Oliver James Garden • John Wong
Editors

General Principles of Surgery

Handbooks in General Surgery

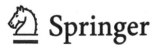 Springer

Editors

Kirby I. Bland, MD
Fay Fletcher Kerner Professor
and Chairman
Department of Surgery
Deputy Director
Comprehensive Cancer Center
University of Alabama School
of Medicine
Birmingham, AL, USA

Markus W. Büchler, MD
Professor of Surgery
and Chairman
Department of General
and Visceral Surgery
University of Heidelberg
Heidelberg, Germany

Attila Csendes, MD, FACS (Hon)
Professor of Surgery
and Chairman
Department of Surgery
University Hospital
Santiago, Chile

Michael G. Sarr, MD
James C. Mason Professor
of Surgery
Department of Surgery
Mayo Clinic College of
Medicine
Rochester, MN, USA

O. James Garden, MBChB, MD,
FRCS (Ed), FRCP (Ed),
FRACS (Hon)
Regius Professor of Clinical
Surgery
Department of Clinical
and Surgical Sciences
The University of Edinburgh
Royal Infirmary of Edinburgh
Edinburgh, UK

John Wong, BSc (Med (Syd)),
MBBS (Syd),
PhD (Syd), MD
(Hon (Syd)),
FRACS, FRCS (Edin),
FRCS (Glasg), FACS (Hon)
Chair Professor
Department of Surgery
The University of Hong Kong
Queen Mary Hospital
Hong Kong, China

ISBN 978-1-84996-380-0   e-ISBN 978-1-84996-381-7

DOI 10.1007/978-1-84996-381-7

Springer London Dordrecht Heidelberg New York

British Library Cataloguing in Publication Data

A catalogue record for this book is available from the British Library

Library of Congress Control Number: 2010933602

Printed on acid-free paper

Springer is part of Springer Science+Business Media (www.springer.com)

ISBN 978-1-84996-380-0   e-ISBN 978-1-84996-381-7

DOI 10.1007/978-1-84996-381-7

Springer London Dordrecht Heidelberg New York

British Library Cataloguing in Publication Data

A catalogue record for this book is available from the British Library

Library of Congress Control Number: 2010933602

Printed on acid-free paper

Springer is part of Springer Science+Business Media (www.springer.com)

Preface

The editors designed the original textbook, *General Surgery: Principles and International Practice,* from which this shorter paperback monograph on the general principles of surgery was taken to be an accessible, concise, and state-of-the-art volume that explores and documents evolutionary principles in the practice of surgery. This work is aimed at the general surgeon and the resident in training. The scientific community continues to witness extraordinary advances in the therapy of both benign and malignant surgical diseases of various organ sites. Much of this progress has been evident over the past decade with new concepts and techniques of management that allow the surgeon to integrate this discipline with medicine, pharmacology, immunology, biostatistics, pathology, genetics, medical and radiation oncology, and diagnostic radiology and imaging. Further, each of these major disciplines contributes a small component for the diagnostic and therapeutic approaches to clinical care; hence the comprehensive planning, integration, and provision of patient care throughout the preoperative, intraoperative, and postoperative phases of care remains essential in the successful practice of our specialty.

The editors acknowledge that the aim of this work is to provide an illustrative, instructive, and comprehensive review that depicts the rationale of basic operative principles essential to surgical therapy. In organizing this monograph, the editors chose authors renowned in the disciplines for illustrating, forming, and depicting in a comprehensive fashion the surgical therapy expectant for metabolic, infectious, endocrine, and neoplastic abnormalities in adult and pediatric patients **from a truly international and multi-continental perspective.** The editors and authors were chosen carefully from across geographies and also from multi-cultural and diverse locations. While the authors consider this text to be inclusive regarding the technical and operative conditions for perioperative care in this field, its purpose should not be intended to replace standard textbooks of surgery nor should it be considered complete in its coverage of pathophysiologic disorders. In contrast, this monograph is organized to familiarize practicing surgeons, residents, and fellows with state-of-the-art surgical principles and techniques essential to contemporary practice. Therefore, the tenor of this monograph on the general principles of surgery has been developed to coexist with other major surgical reference texts that are dedicated—some in more comprehensive fashion—to the therapy of individual organs of systemic diseases. Along with this monograph, nine other paperback monographs are available and focus on surgery in trauma, critical care, esophagus and stomach, small bowel, colorectal, liver and biliary, pancreas and spleen, oncology, and endocrine organs, all adapted from the primary textbook—*General Surgery: Principles and International Practice.*

The chapters in this monograph on the general principles of surgery include a condensed bibliography of highly selective journal articles, reviews, and text. In this manner of attempting to be concise, we hope to provide a precise focus for the education of the reader relative to accepted surgical principles involved in patient care. Moreover, the editors have sought to provide a counterpoint view for the selection of therapy by presenting at the opening of each chapter a list of "Pearls and Pitfalls" that highlight particular concerns or controversies. The chapters provide pertinent, though not exhaustive, summaries of anatomy and physiology, a history of surgical illness, and stages of operative approaches with relevant technical considerations outlined in an easily understandable manner. Complications are reviewed when appropriate for the organ system, diseases, and problem. The text is supported amply by line drawings and photographs that depict anatomic or technical principles. The editors have made every attempt to minimize duplicative or repetitive discussions except when controversial or state-of-the-art issues are presented. Moreover, the editors have attempted to ensure that accurate presentations and illustrations depict properly the most complex problems confronted by the general surgeon.

Finally, in an attempt to address advances in contemporary concepts, the text has been organized to address in detail expeditious, safe, and anatomically accurate operations and incorporate standard as well as evolving surgical principles and techniques. These principles have been tested in the clinics of valid scientific knowledge and are well supported by the time-tested approaches that have been provided by practicing surgeons. The editors are excited to be able to respond to the challenge of developing a truly international text and are indeed hopeful that our readers will find this focused monograph on the general principles of surgery to be a repository of insight, useful, and timely information.

Kirby I. Bland
Michael G. Sarr
Markus W. Büchler
Attila Csendes
O. James Garden
John Wong

Contents

Contributors

Walter L. Biffl, MD, FACS
Associate Professor, Department of Surgery,
Denver Health Medical Center/University of
Colorado-Denver, Denver, CO, USA

William G. Cioffi, MD, FACS
Professor and Chair, Department of Surgery,
Brown Medical School, Providence, RI, USA

Henry M. Cryer, MD, PhD, FACS
Professor in Surgery, Chief of Trauma and Critical Care,
Department of Surgery, David Geffen School of Medicine at
UCLA, Los Angeles, CA, USA

Kimberly A. Davis, MD, FACS
Associate Professor of Surgery, Department of Surgery,
Yale University School of Medicine, New Haven, CT, USA

**Kenneth C.H. Fearon, MBChB, MD, FRCPS (Glas),
FRCPS(Ed), FRCPS(Eng)**
Professor of Surgical Oncology, University of Edinburgh,
Royal Infirmary of Edinburgh, Edinburgh, UK

Richard L. Gamelli, MD, FACS
Robert J. Freeark Professor and Chairman,
Department of Surgery, Loyola University Medical Center,
Maywood, IL, USA

W. Scott Jellish, MD, PhD
Professor, Department of Anesthesiology,
Loyola University Medical Center, Maywood, IL, USA

Eric J. Mahoney, MD
Instructor, Department of Surgery, Brown Medical School,
Providence, RI, USA

Mary C. McCarthy, MD
Professor, Division of Trauma, Critical Care, and
Emergency Surgery, Department of Surgery,
Wright State University, Boonshoft School of Medicine,
Dayton, OH, USA

Edmund A.M. Neugebauer, PhD
Director and Chairman for Surgical Research,
Faculty of Medicine, Institute for Research in Operative
Medicine, University Witten/Herdecke, Cologne, Germany

Richard J.E. Skipworth, BSc(Hons), MBChB, MRCS(Ed)
Clinical Research Fellow, University of Edinburgh Royal
Infirmary of Edinburgh, Edinburgh, UK

Randy J. Woods, MD
Assistant Professor, Division of Trauma, Critical Care,
and Emergency Surgery, Department of Surgery,
Wright State University School of Medicine,
Miami Valley Hospital, Dayton, OH, USA

1
Anesthesia and Risk Management

W. Scott Jellish

Pearls and Pitfalls

- An adequate review of systems is key to determining physical health and providing an assessment of perioperative risk. A few extra minutes spent obtaining an adequate history will reduce the ordering and expense of unnecessary tests.
- The value of exercise tolerance and the ability to accomplish 4 metabolic equivalents (METS) of activity can be used to predict complication rates for many surgeries.
- The ability to intubate and ventilate a patient is of primary importance and weighs heavily on the assessment of risk.
- Electrocardiograms (ECGs) are useful, not as a screening tool, but as a modality for obtaining a more accurate medical assessment of patients in high-risk groups.
- Avoid the technology trap. Nonselective batteries of tests will often

  - Fail to uncover pathologic conditions
  - Detect abnormalities that do not necessarily improve outcome
  - Increase medicolegal liability because of poor follow-up

- Low serum albumin is a marker of increased pulmonary complications and should be measured in all patients suspected of poor diet or hypoalbuminemia.

K.I. Bland et al. (eds.), *General Principles of Surgery*,
DOI 10.1007/978-1-84996-381-7_1,
© Springer-Verlag London Limited 2011

- A patient's emotional and psychiatric needs are as important as physical status in assessing perioperative risk and post-operative outcome. These variables should be thoroughly evaluated.

Risk assessment by the anesthesiologist is a complex task incorporating numerous physical and laboratory findings. Physical status and the ability of the patient to withstand the stress of the surgical procedure must be determined. The assess-ment of risk is based on the knowledge of prevalence rates of unwanted consequences in population groups sharing the same characteristics or risk factors. The preoperative interview should educate the patients about anesthesia perioperative care and pain treatment to reduce anxiety and facilitate recovery. The complex interaction between perceived risk, benefit, and the acceptance of that risk is influenced by charac-teristics such as familiarity, control, catastrophe potential, and level of knowledge. Medical counseling during the presurgical assessment is used to obtain pertinent information about the patient's medical history, as well as physical and mental condi-tion. The care plan is determined and guided by patient choices, which helps relieve anxiety and establish mutual trust.

Important Goals For Preoperative Preparation Prior to Surgery

Risk management involves identification of risk and either avoiding conditions which predispose the patient to that risk, or developing a means to alter the consequences of an action or event which usually leads to an adverse outcome. Factors that affect risk include: the nature and duration of the illness requiring the operation, other comorbidities, age, nutritional status, as well as the type of operation consid-ered. The American Society of Anesthesiologists Task Force on Preanesthesia Evaluation issued a Practice Advisory which focuses on the timing of the evaluation, choice of tests, and the recommendation that no tests beyond a physician evaluation be ordered for patients undergoing minimally invasive surgical procedures. It is the task of the anesthesiologist to assess risk and formulate an acceptable plan which will anticipate potential problems, increase patient safety, produce an acceptable operating field, and provide a stable and pain-controlled postoperative environment.

The preoperative assessment is based on a thorough and efficient fact-finding process. The ultimate goals are to reduce the morbidity associated with surgery, increase the quality, decrease the costs of perioperative care, and restore the patient quickly to their preoperative level of functionality. This assessment includes decisions for noninvasive testing to better estimate risk and determine patients who might benefit from specific preoperative procedures. Indirect studies of perioperative morbidity over four decades have shown that perioperative patient conditions are significant predictors of postoperative morbidity. The fact finding methods used by anesthesiologists to assess surgical risk include: an adequate history, physical exam, and finally, confirmatory laboratory tests as directed by the history and physical exam. This not only improves outcomes but also reduces costs. It is the medical history that will give the most information concerning the patient and their ability to undergo the surgical procedure. The history has been demonstrated to give primary information concerning a patient's physical state in approximately 60% of cases. It should include both acute and chronic aspects of the patients health and should be focused on the upcoming surgical procedure. The first key aspect of the acute history is exercise tolerance. Patients are usually asked if they can climb two flights of stairs, which is 4 METS of activity. An inability to perform 4 METS of activity should arouse suspicion of congestive heart failure or coronary disease. The METS criteria are primarily based on studies that found that the complication rate for noncardiac surgery in elderly patients doubled if they were unable to complete 4 METS of activity. Other studies have demonstrated that the 4 METS rule can be used to predict complication rates in vascular and bariatric surgery, among others. Information concerning medications is the second key consideration and includes questions about supplements and why they are taken. Questions determining vitality, mobility, and fitness are also asked, along with a review of systems focusing on chronic disease, history of hospitalization and surgeries, family history, and social history.

A major factor that is always considered in a patient undergoing surgery is age. Although much of the increased morbidity related to age is appropriately attributable to comorbidity and the extent of the existing disease, a patient >80 years of age will have a reduced physiologic reserve. Numerous studies have found a significant increase in mortality after surgery beginning at the age of 70. The highest rate of anesthetic complications occurs in an age group >75 and among those with the greatest number of comorbidities. Thirty six percent of patients over 70 had nonfatal complications after surgery. In patients undergoing vascular procedures, the single best predictor of death, pulmonary edema, cardiac arrest, or myocardial infarction was age >70.

To assess operative risk, the anesthesiologist must also include a physical examination of the patient. In most instances, pertinent physical findings have already been established by the primary care or general medicine physician. However, there are some instances where the anesthesiologist discovers a previously undiagnosed finding (murmur, bruit, etc.) that may require further investigation. There are a few physical features that are important to the anesthesiologist which directly affect intraoperative risk, namely the anatomy of the airway and the body habitus of the patient, as it pertains to the anatomical features which could increase the difficulty of a regional anesthetic.

The ability to intubate and ventilate a patient for a surgical procedure is of primary importance to the anesthesiologist and weighs heavily in the assessment of risk criteria. Closed claims analysis reveals that 85% of airway-related incidents involve brain damage or death, and as many as one-third of deaths attributable solely to anesthesia have been related to the inability to maintain a patent airway. Numerous complications and morbidities are associated with endotracheal intubation (Table 1.1). Malformations of the face, acromegaly, cervical

TABLE 1.1. Complications of endotracheal intubation (Reprinted from Mallampati, 1997. With permission).

During intubation	Evident after extubation
Laryngospasm	Laryngospasm
Laceration, bruising of lips, tongue and pharynx	Aspiration of secretions, gastric contents, blood or foreign bodies
Fracture, chipping, dislodgement of teeth or dental appliances	Glottic, subglottic or uvular edema
Perforation of trachea or esophagus	Dysphonia, aphonia
Retropharyngeal dissection	Paralysis of vocal cords or hypoglossal, lingual nerves
Fracture or dislocation of cervical spine	Sore throat
Trauma to eyes	Noncardiogenic pulmonary edema
Hemorrhage	Laryngeal incompetence
Bacteremia	Soreness, dislocation of jaw
Aspiration of gastric contents or foreign bodies	Tracheomalacia
Endobronchial or esophageal intubation	Glottic, subglottic or tracheal stenosis
Dislocation of arytenoid cartilages or mandible	Vocal cord granulomata or synechiae
Hypoxemia, hypercarbia	
Bradycardia, tachycardia	
Hypertension	
Increased intracranial or intraocular pressure	

With tube in situ

Accidental extubation

Endobronchial intubation

Obstruction or kinking

Bronchospasm

Ignition of tube by laser device or cautery

Aspiration

Sinusitis

Excoriation of nose or mouth

spondylosis, occipito-atlanto-axial disease, tumors of the airway, and long-term diabetes producing stiff joint syndrome carry added risk. Head movement and the ability to hyperextend the neck producing a thyromental distance of >6.5 cm would be consistent with a normal airway and easy mask ventilation. The ability of the patient to prognath the jaw and an inter-incisor gap of >5 cm would provide evidence of a large mouth opening which is suggestive of an easy laryngoscopy. Tooth morphology, especially "buck" teeth, may make the intubation extremely difficult. Loose teeth should also be identified as they could become easily dislodged and aspirated during intuba-tion, adding considerable morbidity to the surgical procedure.

The visibility of the oropharyngeal structures is assessed in the sitting position without phonation. Mallampati constructed a staging system to predict difficult tracheal intubation. This system was modified by El Ganzouri et al. to further estimate the success rate of intubation. A Class I designation is made when faucial pillars, soft palate, and uvula are visualized and would be consistent with a normal-appearing airway. Visualization of the faucial pillars and soft palate with an obstructed view of the uvula by the base of the tongue is consistent with a Class II airway. This designation is also considered low-risk for laryngos-copy and intubation. The Class III airway is characterized by visualization of the soft palate only and carries a higher risk for difficult intubation. The Class IV airway with visualization of the hard palate only is considered the most difficult to intubate and carries the highest risk of perioperative morbidity. Any patient diagnosed as having obstructive sleep apnea or in whom it is suspected on the basis of clinical signs (obesity, limited mouth opening, or a large tongue) should be treated as having a diffi-cult airway until proven otherwise.

The next major anesthetic assessment of perioperative risk involves the cardiovascular system and the patient's fitness to undergo the procedure without major morbidity and mortality. The type and duration of surgery, particularly the risk of large blood loss, volume shifts, violation of visceral cavities, or vascular procedures, account for major surgical procedures with the greatest potential for complications (Table 1.2). In addition, certain timing factors may influence the risk of the surgical

TABLE 1.2. Cardiac risk stratification for noncardiac surgical procedures[a] (Reproduced from ACC/AHA Guideline Update for Perioperative Cardiovascular Evaluation for Non-Cardiac Surgery – Executive Summary, 2002, American Heart Association. With permission).

Stratification

High (reported cardiac risk often >5%)

Emergent major operations, particularly in the elderly

Aortic and other major vascular procedures

Peripheral vascular procedures

Anticipated prolonged surgical procedures associated with large fluid shifts and/or blood loss

Intermediate (reported cardiac risk generally <5%)

Carotid endarterectomy

Head and neck procedures

Intraperitoneal and intrathoracic procedures

Orthopedic procedures

Prostate surgery

Low[b] (reported cardiac risk generally <1%)

Endoscopic procedures

Superficial procedure

Cataract removal

Breast procedures

[a]*Cardiac risk signifies combined incidence of cardiac death and nonfatal myocardial infarction.*
[b]*Does not generally require further preoperative testing.*

procedure. Cardiac complications are 2–5 times more likely to occur with surgeries in the emergency setting than when done electively (Mozaffarian, 2005). Patients presenting for cardiac procedures (bypass, valve replacement, etc.) assume a higher risk of cardiac-related morbidity and mortality by the nature of their surgery.

The patient that presents for noncardiac surgery poses the biggest problem for the assessment of fitness to undergo a surgical procedure. History-taking alone often provides enough information to determine a patient's risk of complications for the proposed surgery. Questions directed toward the occurrence of any previous myocardial infarction and the presence and frequency of any precipitating or potentiating factors involving any chest discomfort, may be an indication of ischemia. Questions should also be directed towards symptoms of heart failure (orthopnea, paroxysmal nocturnal dyspnea, and dyspnea on exertion) and the results of previous cardiac tests. The physical exam should include the measurement of vital signs and evidence of peripheral vascular disease (carotid or femoral bruits or diminished pulses). The lung fields should be examined for decreased breath sounds, rales, or rhonchi.

The patient with a suspicious history who has symptoms or physical evidence of unstable angina, congestive heart failure, or rhythm disturbances is at high risk for a myocardial event. High-cardiac risk patients need further investigation to determine functional status or if the degree of myocardial ischemia will be altered by subsequent therapy. The additional diagnostic procedures performed in high- or intermediate-risk patients help the anesthesiologist determine the extent of intraoperative monitoring, the anesthetic plan, and even if the procedure should be avoided altogether.

An ECG sometimes uncovers occult disease in older adults, but it rarely shows clinically important abnormalities in younger asymptomatic patients without cardiac risk factors. The usefulness of the preoperative ECG depends on the information it provides physicians to identify cardiac risk, quantify abnormalities in known risk, and make decisions about perioperative therapy. Routine ECGs in asymptomatic women under 50 and men under 40 are usually not indicated.

Patients who benefit from a preoperative ECG manifest one or more of the following conditions: chest pain not ascribed to any etiology, angina or anginal equivalents, history of congestive heart failure, high blood pressure, diabetes or symptoms of dysrhythmias, shortness of breath, history of smoking, inability to exercise, or need for vascular surgery.

Abnormalities on ECG that have the potential to alter management of perioperative care are: atrial flutter or fibrillation; first-, second-, or third-degree AV block; ST segment changes suggestive of myocardial ischemia; premature ventricular and atrial contractions; LV or RV hypertrophy; short P–R interval; Wolf Parkinson-White syndrome; prolonged QT; peaked t waves; and small voltage indicative of cardiomyopathy. The consensus exists that ECGs are useful, not as a screening tool, but as a tool for obtaining a more accurate medical assessment of patients in otherwise high-risk groups.

Further cardiac studies to stratify risk may be most beneficial for patients who are considered to be at intermediate risk of cardiac complications. These tests may also be indicated for patients with known or suspected coronary artery disease who are undergoing high-risk procedures and in whom functional status and stability of ischemia is difficult to assess. Testing the low-risk patient undergoing low-risk surgery is an exercise in futility. There are some generally accepted principles regarding what exactly is an effective screening test. It must be accurate and able to detect the target condition earlier than without screening and with efficient accuracy to avoid producing large amounts of false-positive or false-negatives. The test should improve the likelihood of favorable health outcomes compared to treating patients once they present with signs or symptoms of the disease. The threshold for ordering these tests should reflect the cardiac risk of the planned procedure.

The ECG exercise treadmill test is useful in patients who can exercise but is rarely applicable to patients with ischemic lower extremities. Studies have demonstrated that standard exercise stress tests were falsely positive for significant coronary artery disease in 40% of patients and falsely negative in 15%. Many times, the patient cannot achieve the maximum predicted heart rate because of dyspnea or claudication. Thus in a population with a high prevalence of coronary artery disease, a positive exercise stress test only slightly increases the likelihood of coronary artery disease and a negative test correlates poorly with the absence of heart disease. Therefore interest has increased in other noninvasive tests for cardiac risk stratification.

Holter monitoring or ambulatory ECG for detecting asymptomatic ischemia is not widely used, but its findings may correlate well with those of exercise testing and dipyridamole-thallium scans (DTS) in predicting adverse cardiac events. The ST changes indicative of ischemia (1 mm ST depression for at least 1 min) often can be seen at heart rates below those obtained by conventional stress testing. Several studies have concluded that ischemia detected during Holter monitoring was a reliable predictor of postoperative cardiac events even after all other risk factors were controlled. Comparisons of exercise tolerance tests, Holter monitoring, and cardiac catheterization in patients with stable angina revealed that patients with positive Holter results had a greater likelihood of having multi-vessel coronary artery disease. The advantages of Holter monitoring to identify high-risk patients for cardiac complications include its availability, ease of interpretation, and low cost. However, it is used the least in clinical practice to assess perioperative risk. It is of no value in patients with pre-existing ECG abnormalities that obfuscate determinations of ST segment depression.

Pharmacological stress testing should be considered for patients with an abnormal ECG (including left and possibly right bundle branch block and a history of myocardial infarction). It should also be considered for those taking digoxin and in those who cannot exercise to acceptable levels. As with all tests, their predictive value to determine adverse cardiac outcome is important. Relative risk is the probability of an adverse event where the test is negative. A high score determines a high risk of a cardiac event, whereas a score of 1 implies that risk is similar whether the test is positive or negative. Relative risk scores have been developed for noninvasive cardiac tests and help determine the effectiveness of these tests for prediction of poor outcome. Studies of cardiac risk using DTS suggest that patients with normal studies have a low risk for cardiac complications (good negative predictive value); however, the prognostic implications of an abnormal scan are less well established. Prospective studies to determine the efficacy of DTS on predicting intraoperative myocardial ischemia or infarct suggest a close relationship between reversible defects and adverse cardiac outcome. The sensitivity of the exam, however, appears to be in the presence or absence of coronary artery disease, but not ischemia. The combined median relative risk score for this test was 4.6. However, recent reports demonstrate no correlation between redistribution defects and adverse cardiac outcome or risk of perioperative ischemia. Thus routine DTS screening is not recommended for determination of adverse cardiac outcome.

Radionucleide ventriculography (RNVG) and assessment of left ventricle function and ejection fraction (EF) can predict perioperative cardiac morbidity in patients undergoing vascular procedures. In addition to determining EF, the scan can show ventricular wall motion abnormalities and systolic and diastolic dysfunction. Pasternak et al. demonstrated that a calculated EF of less than 35% was associated with a perioperative myocardial infarction rate of 20%. The combined relative risk with this stipulated EF was 3.7, delineating a positive result. Although not all studies have substantiated the accuracy of RNVG for predicting postoperative cardiac mortality, measurement of EF using this technique is one of the strongest predictors of overall and late survival after vascular surgery.

Dobutamine stress echo (DSE) was developed as a tool for assessing the presence of coronary artery disease. The exam is composed of the administration of a pharmacologic inotropic agent (dobutamine) which increases heart rate and myocardial contractility, thereby increasing myocardial oxygen (O_2) consumption. If O_2 demand outstrips supply, myocardial dysfunction will be evident by echocardiographic evidence of hypokinesis, akinesis, or dyskinesis. The development of new wall motion abnormalities following dobutamine is considered indicative of significant heart disease. This test is recommended in patients with intermediate clinical predictors (prior MI, compensated CHF, diabetes, and mild angina) with poor functional capacity (<4 METS) or intermediate clinical predictors with moderate or excellent functional capacity (>4 METS) and high surgical risk. DSE and DTS appear to have comparable specificity and sensitivity; however, relative risk scores generated from numerous outcome studies were demonstrated to average 6.2 for DSE, which suggests the test may be more effective for predicting an adverse cardiac event.

Coronary artery plaque burden and coronary calcium evaluation using electron beam computed tomography (EBCT) has recently been touted to be diagnostic for coronary artery disease risk. The test examines coronary plaque burden and found that those with coronary calcium scores >1,000 all had elevation of cardiac troponin-T perioperatively. However, EBCT's ability to reduce morbidity and mortality has not been demonstrated, and more importantly, the cost-effectiveness and consequences of negative tests and false-positives are unknown. Thus it is not recommended as a screening tool for perioperative cardiac morbidity.

Coronary angiography is not recommended for risk assessment in patients going for noncardiac surgery unless they have clinical evidence of coronary artery disease and are undergoing moderate- to high-risk surgical procedures. If coronary artery disease or cardiac dysfunction is severe enough to request coronary angiography, the anesthesiologist presumes the risk to be high and the patient in question will undergo a cardiac event during surgery. The anesthesiologist also presumes a coronary artery bypass graft (CABG) or percutaneous transluminal coronary angioplasty (PTCA) will be performed if appropriate lesions are found. The presence of significant coronary stenosis does not always indicate that an MI is unavoidable or that invasive monitoring is required because the involved artery may supply a scar or its stenosis may be compensated by collaterals. The use of coronary angiography to assess risk for perioperative morbidity and mortality is not supported at present and studies to evaluate its use are ongoing.

The evaluation of pulmonary function is also important in assessing patient risk for surgery. In fact, recent recommendations from the American College of Physicians stress that patients be evaluated for the presence of the following risk factors for postoperative pulmonary complications: chronic obstructive pulmonary disease, age >60 years, ASA physical status II or greater, functional dependence, and congestive heart failure (Roizen, 1993). Obesity and mild or moderate asthma were not significant risk factors. Pulmonary complications are the most common form of postoperative morbidity expressed by patients who undergo abdominal and thoracic procedures. In addition to pneumonia, postoperative pulmonary complications include massive lobar collapse due to mucous plugging, pneumonitis, atelectasis, and a combination of one or more of these problems. The high incidence of these complications and their associated costs make it imperative that patients at increased risk be identified and pulmonary function optimized prior to the surgical procedure. The anesthesiologist may request pulmonary function tests to assess risk prior to intrathoracic procedures to determine if the patient will tolerate loss of functional lung units. The calculation of percent predicted volume has increased the accuracy of spirometry as a preoperative tool for evaluating pulmonary risk. The risk assessment by the anesthesiologist will also include methods to reduce pain and techniques to preserve viable lung function postoperatively.

Abdominal procedures produce a 30% incidence of pulmonary complications. In addition to dysfunction of the abdominal musculature, abdominal surgery impairs diaphragmatic function, which further reduces FRC. The preoperative evaluation of pulmonary risk in the patient undergoing abdominal surgery should include age, general health performance, weight, coexisting pulmonary morbidity and the type and approach for the surgery. Spirometry is indicated in patients in whom severe pulmonary dysfunction is evident as a means to assess whether they may need pulmonary rehabilitation prior to surgery. Other procedures that have a high risk of pulmonary complications include prolonged surgeries (>3 h), neurosurgery, head and neck surgery, vascular surgery, emergency surgery, and aortic aneurysm repair.

A low serum albumin (<3.5 g/dl) is also a marker of increased risk for postoperative pulmonary complications and should be measured in all patients who are clinically suspected of hypoalbuminemia. Other tests have also been suggested to estimate pulmonary risk. Spirometry diagnoses obstructive lung disease but does not translate into an effective risk predictor for patients. Comparisons of spirometric studies with clinical data have not consistently demonstrated it to be superior to history and physical exams in predicting postoperative pulmonary complications. Chest radiographs are frequently used as part of a routine preoperative evaluation of risk. The evidence suggests, however, that clinicians may predict most abnormal preoperative chest radiographs by history and physical exams and that this test only rarely provides unexpected information. Chest radiographs are helpful for patients with known cardiopulmonary disease and those older than 50 who are undergoing upper abdominal, thoracic, or abdominal aortic aneurysm surgery.

The numerous factors considered in the perioperative assessment of risk make exchange of information sometimes difficult and hard to convey. A generalized scoring system of risk allows groups of patients to be stratified according to the severity of their illness before treatment is begun and enables better analysis of morbidity and mortality for these groups. A risk scoring system should have several prerequisites: (1) simple to use; (2) applicable to most general surgery cases; (3) used for both elective and emergency procedures; and (4) universally accepted to assess both morbidity and mortality. The scoring system most often used by anesthesiologists to assess risk is the American Society of Anesthesiologists Physical Status classification. Patients are allocated to one of five categories based on their medical history and physical examination without the use of any specific tests. A physical status I (PS I) designates a normal healthy patient while a PS IV individual has incapacitating disease that limits lifestyle and is a threat to life. PS V patients are moribund and not expected to survive more than 24 h. An "E" designation is added to denote an emergency procedure with an associated increase in risk. Postoperative morbidity and mortality rise with increased ASA grade, and if age is added as a covariable, the scoring system has an even better predictive effect (Table 1.3).

TABLE 1.3. American Society of Anesthesiologists Classification (Qaseem et al., 2006).

ASA class	Rates of PPCs class definition by class (%)
I A normally healthy patient	1.2
II A patient with mild systemic disease	5.4
III A patient with systemic disease that is not incapacitating	11.4
IV A patient with an incapacitating systemic disease that is a constant threat to life	10.9
V A moribund patient who is not expected to survive for 24 h with or without operation	N/A

ASA = American Society of Anesthesiologists; NA = not applicable; PPC = postoperative pulmonary complication.

TABLE 1.4. Goldman's nine independent variables associated with perioperative cardiac events (Data from Goldman et al., 1977).

Age over 70 years

Myocardial infarction in the preceding 6 months

Perioperative third heart sound or jugular venous distention

Significant valvular aortic stenosis

Emergency surgery

Intraperitoneal, intrathoracic, or aortic operation

More than five premature ventricular beats per minute documented at any time before operation

Rhythm other than sinus or the presence of atrial premature contractions on preoperative electrocardiogram

One or more markers of poor general medical condition

The Goldman Cardiac Risk Index was designed to predict the risk of cardiac complications following noncardiac surgery. Nine factors are considered to give a total score of 0–53 (Table 1.4) Scores are then grouped into four risk classes. Originally, Goldman was critical of the ASA classification system as being poorly defined and subjective, but it has proved to be as good as the more cumbersome Goldman classification which is not routinely used today by anesthesiologists. Other classification systems, such as the Pulmonary Complication Risk and the Prognostic Nutritional Risk scoring systems are used to determine operative risk based on prolonged preoperative hospitalizations of debilitated patients. These scoring systems are too wide-ranging and not specific enough to be used as the basis for individual decision-making concerning the patient about to undergo surgery and are rarely used by anesthesiologists.

Once the assessment of operative risk has been determined the anesthesiologist should also make specific recommendations concerning the discontinuation of oral intake and the reduction of aspiration risk. Metoclopramide, ranitidine, and sodium citrate may be given prior to the scheduled surgery to reduce the risk of aspiration, especially if the patient has a condition which predisposes them to passive reflux of stomach contents (e.g. hiatal hernia, gastroesophageal reflux disease). If the airway is judged acceptable to proceed with direct laryngoscopy, cricoid pressure is used and a rapid sequence induction performed to obtain a patent airway. These procedures done correctly will reduce the risk of aspiration and the accompanying increase in morbidity and mortality associated with such an occurrence.

The physical and mental state of the anesthesiologist is another variable, though not assessed at the time of the preoperative visit that affects the overall risk of the surgical procedure. Human errors affect patient safety in two ways: (1) they increase the probability of accident initiators; and (2) they increase the probability of a failure to properly respond to a problem. Anesthesiologists can experience a number of potential problems that could affect patient outcome. Fatigue and sleep deprivation affect vigilance and the recognition of problems as they occur during the operation. Suitability factors may also be present in which the person lacks the appropriate personality, temperament, or ability to perform anesthesia. Cognitive problems occur in which individuals cannot process all of the information presented to them at a particular time. In addition, the individual may try to cut corners or be careless. Detractors in the operating room could also increase risk to the patient. Social conversations, noise, and considerations of upcoming cases may distract the anesthesiologist from events that occur during the surgical procedure, which may lead to increased morbidity. Aging also affects the operating team, in which case the abilities of both the surgeon and anesthesiologist decline. Lack of continuing education and unfamiliarity with new techniques put the older anesthesiologist at a distinct disadvantage when dangerous situations arise. These human factors could ultimately increase the risk of a particular surgical procedure to a much greater extent than predicted by risk assessments obtained from medical history and laboratory testing.

The final portion of the preoperative risk assessment involves the explanation of risk to the patient and their acceptance of the perceived risk. This explanation also includes discussion of the anesthetic plan and agreement of that plan with the patient and surgeon. The assessment of surgical risk is the best guess of what might happen from a combination of past clinical experiences, cohort data from groups of patients with similar problems, and the patient's own comorbidities. Medical counseling and decision-making is largely about handling these risks. However simple the awaited surgical procedure, it is a very important event in the patient's life. Though small, there is a certain level of risk associated with the simplest surgical interventions, and the patient has a legal right to secure information including risk factors that are specific to their particular case. The patient's agreement to undergo the surgical procedure utilizing the anesthetic technique discussed, is perceived as a contract between physician and patient that is governed by mutual trust established during the preoperative visit. At a time when the patient's right to decide his or her own medical management is becoming more prevalent, the preoperative assessment and the estimate of operative risk play a vital role in the informed consent process and is the cornerstone to a successful surgical outcome.

Selected Readings

Archer C, Levy AR, McGreor M (1993) Value of routine perioperative chest x-rays: a meta-analysis. Can J Anaesth 40:1022–1027

Eagle KA, Berger PB, Calkins H, et al. (2002) ACC/AHA guideline update for perioperative cardiovascular evaluation for noncardiac surgery – executive summary: a report of the American College of Cardiology/American Heart Association Task Force on Practice Guidelines (Committee to Update the 1996 Guidelines on Perioperative Cardiovascular Evaluation for Noncardiac Surgery). Circulation 105:1257–1267

El-Ganzouri AR, McCarthy RJ, Tuman KJ, et al. (1996) Preoperative airway assessment: predictive value of a multivariate risk index: Anesth Analg 82:1197–1204

Goldman L, Caldera DL, Nussbaum SR, et al. (1977) Multifactorial index of cardiac risk in noncardiac surgical procedures. N Engl J Med 297:845–850

Kertai MD, Boersma E, Bax JJ, et al. (2003) A meta-analysis comparing the prognostic accuracy of six diagnostic tests for predicting perioperative cardiac risk in patients undergoing major vascular surgery. Heart 89:1327–1334

Mallampati SR (1997) Airway management. In: Barash PG, Cullen BF, Stoelting RF (eds) Clinical anesthesia, 3rd edn. J.B. Lippincott, Philadelphia, PA, p 587

Mozaffarian D (2005) Electron-beam computed tomography for coronary calcium – a useful test to screen for coronary artery disease? JAMA 294(22):2897–2900

Pasternak LR, Arens JF, Caplan RA, et al. (2002) Task force on preanesthesia evaluation. Practice advisory for preanesthesia evaluation: a report by the American Society of Anesthesiologists Task Force on Preanesthesia Evaluation. Anesthesiology 96:485–496

Pasternak PF, Imparato AM, Riles TS, et al. (1985) The value of the radionuclide angiogram in the prediction of perioperative myocardial infarction in patients undergoing lower extremity revascularization procedures. Circulation 72(Suppl II):13–17

Pate-Cornell ME, Lakats LM, Murphy DM, et al. (1997) Anesthesia patient risk: a quantitative approach to organizational factors and risk management options. Risk Analysis 17:511–523

Qaseem A, Snow V, Fitterman N, et al. (2006) Risk assessment for and strategies to reduce perioperative pulmonary complications for patients undergoing noncardiothoracic surgery: a guideline from the American College of Physicians. Ann Intern Med 144:575–580

Reilly DF, McNeely MJ, Doerner D, et al. (1999) Selfreported exercise tolerance and the risk of serious perioperative complications. Arch Intern Med 159:2185–2192

Roizen MF (1993) The usefulness of the perioperative electrocardiogram. J Clin Monit 9:101–103

Sgura FA, Kopecky SL, Grill JP, et al. (2000) Supine exercise capacity identifies patients at low risk for perioperative cardiovascular events and predicts long-term survival. Am J Med 108:334–336

Srinivas M, Roizen MF, Barnard J, et al. (1994) Relative effectiveness of four preoperative tests for predicting adverse cardiac outcomes after vascular surgery: a metaanalysis. Anesth Analg 79:422–433

2

Fluids and Electrolytes

Kimberly A. Davis and Richard L. Gamelli

Pearls and Pitfalls

- Total body water accounts for 60% of body weight – 40% as the intracellular compartment and 20% as the extracellular compartment
- 5% of body weight is the intravascular compartment.
- In adults, daily maintenance volume is 25–30 ml/kg containing about 1 mEq/kg sodium and 1/2 mEq/kg potassium.
- Volume deficit is the most common fluid disorder in the surgical patient.
- All fluid losses are isotonic except for urine and sweat/ evaporation, thus most replacement fluids should be isotonic.
- Isotonic fluid losses are due most commonly to vomiting, diarrhea, nasogastric suctioning, gastrointestinal fistulae, and sequestration of fluids in soft tissue injuries and infections.
- Hyponatremia may result from SIADH (or the syndrome of inappropriate secretion of antidiuretic hormone) related to head trauma; correction involves free water restriction.
- Hypernatremia from loss of free water from diabetes insipidus or high output renal failure requires a slow correction of serum sodium.

K.I. Bland et al. (eds.), *General Principles of Surgery*,
DOI 10.1007/978-1-84996-381-7_2,
© Springer-Verlag London Limited 2011

- Hyperkalemia from renal failure can be treated by intravenous calcium gluconate, insulin/glucose infusion, potassium exchange resins, and hemodialysis.
- After hemorrhage, fluid and protein move from the interstitium to the plasma, so-called transcapillary plasma refill, resulting in restoration of plasma volume and protein concentration, but with reduced oxygen carrying capacity due to decrease in total red cell mass, i.e., a normovolemic anemia.
- The primary goal of resuscitation is restoration of normal tissue perfusion through volume expansion.
- Ringers lactate is the best fluid for acute resuscitation; hypotonic fluids and those containing glucose should be avoided.
- Inadequate restoration of circulating volume can cause persistent acidosis, systemic inflammatory response syndrome, multiple organ dysfunction system, multi-system organ failure, and even death.

Introduction

The great French physiologist, Claude Bernard, was the first to recognize that human beings lived in two very different environments: the external environment, and the "milieu intérieur," in which the tissues lived. Another 50 years passed before it was known that this internal environment was closely protected by several intrinsic mechanisms. The outcome of these protective mechanisms was termed "homeostasis" by Walter Cannon, a professor of physiology at Harvard. At the crux of this "milieu intérieur" is the maintenance of normal fluid and electrolyte balance.

Administration and replacement of the body's fluid and electrolytes represents a fundamental component of a surgeon's practice. An understanding of the complex mechanisms of homeostasis is necessary, as most diseases and many injuries, including operative trauma, alter the physiology of fluids and electrolytes within the body. Redistribution of body fluids from one compartment to another, as is seen in response to inflammation, infection, and traumatic injury, usually results in a decrease in the volume of circulating extracellular fluid, and subsequent hypoperfusion or "shock". During resuscitation of patients from shock, a strong working knowledge of normal fluid and electrolyte balance is paramount to assure rapid restoration of circulating volume, and the prevention of the untoward sequelae of the systemic inflammatory response syndrome (SIRS) and multisystem organ failure (MSOF).

Distribution of Body Fluids

Roughly 60% of body mass is made up of water, although this percentage varies with age and sex. The total percentage of body water decreases with increasing age, and women tend to have a lower percentage of body water than men. Body water is divided classically into two fluid compartments: the intracellular compartment (two thirds or 40% total body water) and the extracellular compartment (one third or 20% total body water) (Fig. 2.1). The intracellular space is represented predominantly by muscle mass, in which the major cations are magnesium and potassium, buffered by bicarbonate and negatively charged proteins. The extracellular space has sodium and chloride as its main ions and is further subdivided into the plasma (one quarter or 5% of total body water) and

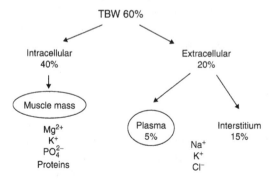

FIGURE 2.1. Body water distribution.

the interstitium (three-quarters or 15% of total body water). Water is freely diffusable across semipermeable membranes, keeping osmotic forces in balance. The forces that drive fluid movement between compartments are the relative Starling forces between the intracellular and extracellular fluid compartments.

Regulation of Normal Homeostasis

Fluid and Electrolyte Balance

The delicate balance of fluid and electrolytes is normally controlled by the kidneys and the neuroendocrine system. Usually, fluid input and output are equal or in balance. When input exceeds output, the term "positive balance" is employed. Conversely, in those patients in whom output exceeds input, the term "negative balance" is applied.

Most intake of water is liquid, with only a third derived from solids, while output is usually classified as either sensible or insensible. Sensible losses are measurable and include urine (800–1,500 ml per day), feces (150 ml per day), and sweat (200–1,000 ml per day). Insensible losses are nonmeasurable and involve evaporation of water from the lungs (exhaled air) and diffusion of water through the skin. Up to 8–12 ml/kg/day is lost through the skin and respiratory tract as insensible loss in the normal human being. Although fairly fixed, insensible loss varies with body temperature, ambient temperature, activity, and daily fluid intake.

The Kidney

Although the type and quantity of input is important, the composition of the "milieu intérieur" is maintained predominantly by the nature of the output; thus the kidneys serve as the primary organ for maintaining constancy of the internal environment. By varying the glomerular filtration rate, the kidneys are able to respond rapidly to changes in volume, solute content and composition of body fluids.

Normal kidney function involves filtration of approximately 180 l of plasma per day. Sodium is resorbed preferentially in the proximal tubule in conjunction with bicarbonate and other divalent cations. The loop of Henle is responsible predominantly for the resorption of water and sodium in conjunction with chloride. In the distal tubule, however, active sodium resorption is coupled with excretion of potassium and hydrogen ion under the control of aldosterone, thus representing a sodium/potassium or sodium/hydrogen exchange. The collecting duct, under the control of ADH (antidiuretic hormone, or arginine vasopressin) results in the resorption of water, and subsequent concentration of the urine. Thus, the maintenance of normal fluid and electrolyte balance is dependent on the formation of a large quantity of glomerular filtrate that is almost completely resorbed from the renal tubules prior to excretion.

Neuroendocrine Control of Renal Function

Changes in fluid and electrolyte balance and renal function normally occur daily as a result of variations in intake and output, or abnormally after injury or illness. Both the volume and composition of body fluids are monitored continuously by receptors and transduced via the neuroendocrine system into changes in renal handling of water and electrolytes. Effective circulating volume is monitored continuously by arterial and renal baroreceptors and by atrial stretch receptors. When effective circulating volume decreases, activity from these receptors decreases, releasing a tonic inhibition from the neuroendocrine system, mediated by increased secretion of adrenocorticotropic hormone (ACTH), resulting in increased aldosterone secretion, and increased secretion of renin, resulting in increased formation of angiotensin. Aldosterone, synthesized, stored, and secreted by the adrenal gland, increases sodium and chloride resorption and potassium excretion in the kidney. Angiotensin, in addition to being a potent vasoconstrictor and myocardial stimulant, stimulates release of ADH, resulting in resorption of free water and augmenting the release of aldosterone. The net effect of these neuroendocrine pathways is to restore circulating volume and maintain normal body fluid and electrolyte balance.

Maintenance of Normal Fluid Balance

Baseline requirements for healthy human beings must account for both insensible losses (approximately 750 ml of pure water per day) and sensible losses of hypotonic fluids of (approximately 350 ml per day). Additionally, a normal person must excrete approximately 600 mOsm per day via the urine to maintain normal body composition secondary to metabolism. The minimal volume of urine necessary to accomplish this varies widely based on the ability of the kidney to concentrate urine, but approximates 500–800 ml per day. Therefore, under normal conditions, the average 70 kg male requires between 1,500 and 2,500 ml of fluid per day, or about 25–30 ml/kg body weight per day (Table 2.1).

The healthy human being also requires a minimal amount of sodium chloride to maintain a normal balance. When human beings are stressed to conserve sodium, they do so at the expense of potassium via the sodium/potassium exchange in the kidney related to aldosterone secretion. Thus, an intake of approximately 60–100 mEq of sodium are necessary per day to prevent excess potassium loss, or approximately 1 mEq/kg

TABLE 2.1. Maintenance fluid requirements for the surgical patient.

Body weight	Fluid requirement
For 0–10 kg	100 ml/kg/day
For 10–20 kg	50 ml/kg/day
For > 20 kg	20 ml/kg/day
For 70 kg adult	2,500 ml/day

body weight. With adequate maintenance doses of sodium, urinary potassium loss will be about 30–60 mEq per day, or approximately 0.5 mEq/kg body weight per day.

Conditions of Abnormal Fluid Loss

Any abnormal fluid losses (replacement) must be added to the daily fluid and electrolyte requirements described above. Most replacement represents losses of transcellular fluids, with varied electrolyte compositions. Normal concentrations found in several body fluids are listed in Table 2.2. Abnormally high secretion of any of these fluids, particularly those from the gastrointestinal tract, is a major cause of fluid and electrolyte disturbances in surgical patients. Knowledge of the electrolyte composition and volume of the body fluid lost is vital in determining replacement therapy. The electrolyte compositions of commonly available replacement fluids are listed in Table 2.3. Common metabolic disturbances from fluid loss and suggested volume replacement are listed in Table 2.4.

TABLE 2.2. Electrolyte compositions of body fluids (mEq/l).

	Na^+	K^+	Cl^-	HCO_3	Volume (ml)	Osmolality (mOsm/l)
Saliva	10	26	10	30	1,000	Variable
Stomach	60[a]	10	130	0	1,500	280
Duodenum	140	5	80	0	1,500	280
Ileum	140	5	104	30	3,000	280
Colon	60	35	40	0	750	280
Pancreas	145	5	75	115	1,000	280
Bile	145	5	100	35	1,000	280
Sweat	50	5	55	0	500	Variable
Blood	140	5	100	24	5,000	280

[a]Varies with acid secretion; in patients with achlorhydria or after acid-secreting inhibition, sodium approaches 130 mEq/l.

TABLE 2.3. Electrolyte composition of replacement fluids (mEq/l).

Solution	pH	Na$^+$	Cl$^-$	K$^+$	Ca^{2+}	Other components	Osmolality (mOsm/l)
Lactate Ringers (LR)	5	130	109	4	3	Lactate	28 mEq/l
NS	4	154	154	0	0		308
D5LR	5	130	109	4	3	Dextrose 50 g/l, l actate 28 mEq/l	560
D5NS	4	154	154	0	0	Dextrose 50 g/l	588
D5.45NS	4	77	77	0	0	Dextrose 50 g/l	434
D5.25NS	4	34	34	0	0	Dextrose 50 g/l	357

TABLE 2.4. Replacement fluids for the management of common metabolic disturbances.

Source of fluid	Metabolic disturbance	Suggested replacement
Gastric	Hypochloremic, hypokalemic metabolic alkalosis	D5NS with 20 mEq/l KCl
Pancreatic	Acidemia, hypoproteinemia	LR (bicarbonate may be supplemented in D5 water)
Small bowel	Hypovolemia	LR
Colon (diarrhea)	Hypokalemic metabolic acidosis	D5NS with 20 mEq/l KCl

One practical approach to addressing abnormal fluid and electrolyte losses divides the types of loss into alterations in volume, concentration, composition and/or distribution.

Alterations in Volume

If isotonic fluid is added to or lost from body fluids, the volume of extracellular fluid is changed. Sudden loss of an isotonic fluid, such as an intestinal fluid, results in an acute decrease in extracellular fluid volume without changing intracellular fluid volume. As long as the osmolarity between the two compartments remains identical, no net movement of fluid from the intracellular to the extracellular space will occur.

In contrast, the sudden loss of circulating blood volume is different than the loss of an isotonic salt solution. Hemorrhage results in decreased cardiac output with the resultant total body ischemia, which cannot be corrected until blood volume is restored. In the absence of transfusion therapy, this correction requires movement of fluid and protein from the interstitium to the plasma, or "transcapillary plasma refill". Transcapillary refill is triggered initially by a fall in capillary hydrostatic pressure, resulting in the movement of protein-free fluid from the interstitium to the plasma space. A second phase involves the movement of protein into the plasma space in support of plasma oncotic pressure. This change restores plasma volume and protein concentration, but with a reduced oxygen carrying capacity due to the decrease in total red cell mass, i.e., a normovolemic anemia. Transcapillary refill can sustain a relatively fixed level of plasma volume, equal to about two-thirds of the initial plasma volume, irrespective of the rate of bleeding. Plasma refill reaches 33% by 30 min after hemorrhage and 50% by 3 h, allowing a fairly rapid restoration of circulating blood volume.

The diagnosis of an abnormal volume status is clinical. Hypovolemia, or volume deficit, is the most common fluid disorder in the surgical patient. Disorders resulting in a loss of isotonic fluid include vomiting, diarrhea, nasogastric suctioning, and gastrointestinal fistulae. Other causes include sequestration of fluids (third spacing) secondary to soft tissue injuries (e.g., trauma, postoperative) and infections, intra-abdominal and retroperitoneal inflammation, intestinal obstruction, and burns. Signs and symptoms of volume deficit include, but are not limited to, altered mental status, hypotension, tachycardia, decreased skin turgor, and hypothermia. Oliguria secondary to renal hypoperfusion is a common barometer of hypovolemia.

Hypervolemia, or volume excess, may be iatrogenic or secondary to cirrhosis, renal failure, or congestive heart failure. Both plasma and interstitial volumes are increased. Symptoms include ascites, pulmonary edema, and peripheral edema.

Alterations in Concentration

If water is added or lost from the extracellular space, the concentration of osmotically active particles will change. In contrast to the intracellular space, in the extracellular space, sodium represents 90% of the osmotically active particles. Therefore, selective changes in total body water are reflected by sodium concentration. A change in the concentration of osmotically active particles will necessitate the movement of water from one compartment to another to restore osmotic balance across membranes.

Hyponatremia (sodium < 130 mEq/l) is associated with free water excess. Symptoms of hyponatremia include central nervous system signs of increased intracranial pressure and tissue edema. It is important to recognize that severe hyponatremia may be associated with oliguric renal failure, which may not be reversible if therapy is delayed. In the surgical patient, acute hyponatremia usually reflects one of two iatrogenic errors. The first is infusion or ingestion of a large volume of free water at a time when high levels of ADH inhibit compensatory diuresis. This setting is most common early in the postoperative period when there may be a high level of ADH in response to pain and anxiety. The second setting occurs with the use of hypotonic fluids to replace isotonic fluid losses. In the trauma patient with a head injury, hyponatremia may herald the development of SIADH, or the "syndrome of inappropriate ADH" secretion. The need for therapy depends on the severity of associated symptoms. Free water restriction can return sodium concentrations toward normal; however, in selected patients, free water restriction is not adequate, and supplementation with salt-containing solutions (and on occasion with hypertonic (3%) sodium chloride) is necessary to return serum sodium levels to normal.

Hypernatremia (sodium > 145 mEq/l) results from excessive free water loss and can be extra-renal or renal in nature. Extra-renal free water loss results from an increase in metabolism from any cause, particularly fever. Evaporative water loss, either through open wounds or through the administration of un-humidified oxygen to hyperventilating patients (particularly those with a tracheostomy), can also result in dehydration and resultant hypernatremia. Hypernatremia can also result from increased renal water loss. High output renal failure due to ischemia/reperfusion damage to the distal tubules and collecting ducts impairs water resorption. Additionally, loss of the ability to release ADH from the central nervous system, such as occurs after some severe head injuries, can impair water resorption (diabetes insipidus). Finally high osmotic loads, due to the iatrogenic administration of mannitol, glycosuria from poorly controlled diabetes, or excess urea from high nitrogen diets, can result in an osmotically driven diuresis with subsequent free water loss.

Treatment of hypernatremia is directed toward restoring normal osmolality of body fluids, carefully and relatively slowly, because the central nervous system tolerates over-vigorous adjustments in sodium concentration poorly. The volume of free water needed to replace a patient's deficit should be calculated from the following formula and replaced over 2–3 days.

$$\text{Free water deficit} = (\text{total body water}) \times ([Na^+ \text{ patient}]/[Na^+ \text{normal}]) - (\text{total body water})$$

Alterations in Composition

The concentration of most other ions in the extracellular space can change without affecting osmolarity. These changes represent alterations only in composition and do not cause fluid shifts. Of particular importance are concentration changes in potassium or in acid-base balance, via changes in hydrogen ions.

The normal intake of potassium per day is 50–100 mEq, and in the absence of hypokalemia, the majority of this intake is secreted in the urine. About 98% of the potassium in the body is located in the intracellular compartment, at concentrations of 150 mEq/l. Although the amount of extracellular potassium is relatively small, normal potassium concentrations are critical for myocardial and neuromuscular function.

Hypokalemia (<3.5 mEq/l) is the most common electrolyte abnormalities in post-surgical patients, resulting from excessive renal secretion, movement of potassium intracellularly, prolonged administration of potassium-free intravenous solutions or nutrition with ongoing obligatory renal losses, and loss via increased gastrointestinal secretions, particularly colonic (i.e. diarrhea). Renal excretion of potassium is increased when large volumes of sodium ion are resorbed via the normal cation exchange mechanisms of the kidney. Potassium requirements after large isotonic volume replacement are increased, probably through the above mechanism. Additionally, potassium becomes very important in acid-base balance, as movement of potassium in or out of the cell occurs in response to changes in hydrogen ion concentration in the blood. Because alkalosis causes net movement of potassium out of cells, severe metabolic alkalosis may exacerbate hypokalemia, as the kidney will compensate for the alkalosis by increasing hydrogen ion resorption at the expense of potassium. Finally, excessive loss of gastrointestinal fluid can result in profound hypokalemia (see Table 2.1).

Symptoms of hypokalemia include muscle weakness, paralytic ileus, and, if severe, cardiac dysrhythmias. Treatment involves potassium replacement, although no more than 40 mEq/l of potassium may be added to intravenous fluids in the absence of electrocardiographic monitoring. Potassium replacement must be undertaken cautiously in patients with acute or chronic renal insufficiency.

Hyperkalemia (>5 mEq/l) is encountered rarely in patients with normal renal function. Most factors in surgical patients that affect potassium metabolism result in excess secretion of potassium and the tendency toward hypokalemia, except in the patient with abnormal renal function, where hyperkalemia can be a serious concern. Symptoms of hyperkalemia include nausea, vomiting, intestinal colic, and diarrhea. Electrocardiographic abnormalities of mild to moderate hyperkalemia include peaked T-waves. Cardiac dysrhythmias occur at concentrations >7 mEq/l and include atrial asystole, with subsequent ventricular tachycardia and/or fibrillation. Temporary suppression of myocardial irritation related to hyperkalemia can be accomplished with the administration of 1 g of 10% calcium gluconate intravenously, and/or by the concomitant administration of glucose and insulin (50 g glucose with 10 units insulin intravenously), which drives potassium intracellularly. Definitive treatment involves cation exchange resins (Kayexalate) or hemodialysis to remove potassium from the patient.

Acid-base balance: The pH of normal body fluids is maintained within a narrow range of 7.37–7.42, which is necessary to maintain normal body functions. This regulation of pH occurs despite a large daily production of both organic and inorganic acids by normal metabolism. Three mechanisms regulate acid-base metabolism: rapid buffering of acids by salts of weak acids (the bicarbonate buffer system), rapid elimination of acids via the lungs (expired CO_2), and slow elimination of acids by the kidneys (renal compensation).

The pH of the extracellular space is a function of the ratio of bicarbonate salt (HCO_3^-) to carbonic acid (H_2CO_3, which in turn is related to the pCO_2). In simple terms, a ratio of 20:1 between bicarbonate and H_2CO_3 will result in a normal pH via an efficient system of buffering. In metabolic acidosis, the concentration of bicarbonate decreases, resulting in a relative excess of carbonic acid. Respiration then rapidly increases, eliminating larger amounts of carbonic acid as water and CO_2, attempting to return the ratio to 20:1. The reverse occurs in a metabolic alkalosis. In contrast, respiratory acidosis and alkalosis are produced by disturbances in ventilation, resulting in a change in pH from normal values of 0.08 for each 10 mmHg change in pCO_2. Compensation is primary renal, but this compensation is relatively slow. In respiratory acidosis (pCO_2 >45 mmHg), chronic renal compensation results in a 3.5 mEq

TABLE 2.5. Common abnormalities of acid-base metabolism.

Acid-base disorder	Defect	Common cause	Serum bicarbonate concentration	Physiologic compensatory mechanism
Metabolic acidosis	Acid gain or base loss	Lactate, diabetes, diarrhea, fistulae, azotemia	Decreased	Pulmonary (rapid)
Metabolic alkalosis	Base gain or acid loss	Vomiting, NG suction, diuretics	Increased	Pulmonary (rapid)
Respiratory acidosis	CO_2 retention (hypoventilation)	Sedation, COPD	Decreased	Renal (slow)
Respiratory alkalosis	Excessive $CO2$ loss (hyperventilation)	Pain, agitation, mechanical ventilation	Increased	Renal (slow)

increase in HCO_3^- for each 10 mmHg increase in pCO_2, but can take up to 72 h to occur fully. Similarly, in respiratory alkalosis ($pCO2 < 35$ mmHg), renal compensation yields a 5 mEq decrease in HCO_3^- for each 10 mmHg decrease in pCO_2. Common abnormalities of acid-base metabolism in the surgical patient and their causes are shown in Table 2.5.

Alterations in Distribution

In the surgical patient, the decrease in circulating volume due to "third space" losses is of particular importance. Third space loss refers to fluid that extravasates into a compartment other than the intracellular or extracellular compartments. Classically, third spacing occurs only with massive ascites, burns, bowel obstruction, peritonitis, and crush injuries. Inflammatory conditions of the abdomen and retroperitoneum, including pancreatitis, also result in significant intraperitoneal fluid and bowel wall edema. The magnitude of fluid loss from these conditions can be difficult to appreciate without the realization that the peritoneum alone has a 1 m2 surface area, such that a slight increase in thickness due to edema and peritonitis will result in a functional loss of several liters of fluid. Similar large volume losses can occur with severe infections of the soft tissue, such as necrotizing fasciitis, with burn wounds, and with severe crush injuries. Finally, sepsis or SIRS can cause a diffuse capillary leak, with a resultant loss of large volumes of intravascular fluids into the interstitium. In all cases, volume resuscitation is the therapy of choice to restore intravascular volume.

Fluid Replacement Therapy

In surgical patients, fluids are used for either maintenance or resuscitation. Because each has a different goal, the composition of and approach to administration of fluids for maintenance or resuscitation are different fundamentally. Maintenance fluids supply the ongoing fluid and electrolyte requirements of the patient. Resuscitative fluids administered to patients in hypovolemic shock should replace existing fluid deficits, as well as ongoing abnormal fluid losses. Initial resuscitative fluids should be isotonic crystalloid solutions, such as normal saline and/or lactated Ringers, administered in bolus form, starting with approximately 30 ml/kg or 2,000 ml in an average-sized adult or 20 ml/kg in a child.

Hypovolemia, or the loss of intravascular volume, results in inadequate perfusion to the tissues of the body, with the resultant inability to supply metabolic demands and remove metabolic wastes. The primary goal of resuscitation, therefore, is to restore normal tissue perfusion rapidly through volume expansion. During resuscitation, administration of fluids containing glucose will result in hyperglycemia, with a resultant osmotic diuresis; because urine output is a measure of adequacy of visceral perfusion, such an osmotic diuresis might be viewed incorrectly as adequate resuscitation, thereby prolonging the shock period. Therefore, glucose-containing fluids should be avoided in the acute resuscitation of the hypovolemic patient.

Lactated Ringers (LR) solution is isotonic, readily available, inexpensive, and does not aggravate pre-existing electrolyte abnormalities. LR administration does not worsen the lactic acidosis normally present in shock. As volume is restored, lactate is mobilized to the liver and metabolized to bicarbonate, leading to a mild metabolic alkalosis 1–2 days after massive resuscitation with LR. In addition, mild to moderate hyponatremia may also occur, because LR has only 130 mEq/l of sodium. Normal saline (NS) is also an effective resuscitation fluid, particularly in patients with head trauma in whom hyponatremia must be avoided. Hypernatremic, hyperchloremic metabolic acidosis is possible after massive resuscitation with NS, particularly in children and in patients with large burns or severe trauma. Resuscitation with hypotonic fluids should be avoided because these fluids dilute the intravascular space and result in an osmotic pressure gradient with a higher osmotic pressure in the interstitial space, drawing water into the interstitium, and the goal of intravascular volume restoration will not be accomplished.

Inadequate restoration of circulating volume can lead to a cascade of related complications, including persistent acidosis, SIRS, MODS, multi-system organ failure, and eventual death. Traditionally, endpoints of resuscitation have been normalization of hemodynamic parameters, restoration of adequate urine output (0.5 ml/kg/h), and return of normal mental status; however, with the understanding that hypoperfusion can exist with normotension, better markers of tissue perfusion have been sought. Monitoring and optimizing oxygen delivery and mixed venous oxygen saturation via use of pulmonary artery catheters will improve outcome after major surgical procedures. Rapid correction of metabolic acidosis with normalization of base deficits after resuscitation from trauma has also improved survival. The adequacy of resuscitation can also be assessed and survival improved by the correction of abnormalities in gastric intramucosal pH (pHi) measured by gastric tonometry. Finally, a renewed interest has developed in the use of non-invasive near infrared absorption spectroscopy in the trauma patient to assess tissue oxygenation (a marker of oxygen transport) at the end-organ level. Although the ideal marker of adequate resuscitation remains elusive, better techniques to monitor specific end-organ perfusion in the future will allow better optimization of resuscitative efforts.

Selected Readings

Drucker WR, Chadwick CDJ, Gann DS (1981) Transcapillary refill in hemorrhage and shock. Arch Surg 116:1344–1353

Elliot DC (1998) An evaluation of endpoints of resuscitation. J Am Coll Surg 187:536–547

Henry S, Scalea TM (1999) Resuscitation in the new millennium. Surg Clin North Am 79(6):1259–1267

Maynard N, Bihari D, Beale R, et al. (1993) Assessment of splanchnic oxygenation by gastric tonometry in patients with acute circulatory failure. JAMA 270:1203–1210

Porter JM, Ivatury RR (1998) In search of the optimal end points of resuscitation in trauma patients: a review. J Trauma 44:908–914

Shoemaker WC, Kram HB, Appel PL (1990) Therapy of shock based on pathophysiology, monitoring and outcome prediction. Crit Care Med 18:S19–S25

3
Nutritional Support in the Surgical Patient

Richard J.E. Skipworth and Kenneth C.H. Fearon

Pearls and Pitfalls

- Manage well-nourished elective patients according to "stress-free" Enhanced Recovery After Surgery (ERAS) principles with optimal pain relief, pro-active management of gut function and early mobilization.
- Allow oral fluids until 2 h prior to operation to decrease dehydration, and consider routine preoperative oral carbohydrate and fluid loading to promote post-operative anabolism.
- Employ thoracic epidural anesthesia to reduce sympathetic activation, prevent paralytic ileus, control pain on movement, and promote mobilization.
- Recommence feeding early in the post-operative period. If voluntary nutritional intake is inadequate, supplement with artificial nutritional support.
- Use enteral nutrition in preference to parenteral nutrition in patients with functioning gastrointestinal (GI) tracts.
- Commence early oral/enteral nutritional support in all malnourished surgical patients to reduce the effects of the stress response and prevent post-operative complications.
- Modern perioperative care means that even if the patient is moderately malnourished, preoperative nutritional support is likely to be of limited benefit. Instead, proceed with surgery and plan for adequate *post-operative* and *post-discharge* nutritional support.

K.I. Bland et al. (eds.), *General Principles of Surgery*,
DOI 10.1007/978-1-84996-381-7_3,
© Springer-Verlag London Limited 2011

- In patients who are severely malnourished, it is often prudent to review the appropriateness of surgical intervention.
- Consider carefully the likely clinical course of a post-operative patient who develops complications. If likely total downtime of gut function from time of surgery is > 5–7 days, always institute artificial nutritional support (especially if the patient has pre-existing malnutrition).

Introduction

Patients undergoing major surgery are at high risk of malnutrition due to the combination of perioperative starvation and activation of both the immune system and the neuroendocrine stress response. Starvation reduces the anabolic substrate available to the patient, whereas the immune/stress response induces whole-body catabolism. In particular, the stress response to surgery and trauma is associated with a significant increase in metabolic rate, glucose and fatty acid utilization, gluconeogenesis, and skeletal muscle protein degradation. These factors all contribute to the depletion of protein, lipid and carbohydrate stores and deterioration in nutritional status. In turn, poor nutritional status is linked with adverse outcome via the effects of tissue wasting and impaired organ function. Loss of power and the increased fatigability of wasted skeletal muscle delays mobilization and affects respiratory and cardiac function, whereas impaired immune function confers increased susceptibility to infection. Thus, malnourished surgical patients are at increased risk of cardio-respiratory embarrassment, chest and wound infections, prolonged hospitalization and death.

Maintenance/optimization of nutritional status is an integral component of standard surgical and trauma care. Nutritional supplementation for surgical patients, if administered appropriately, can be shown to enhance outcome and improve patient quality of life in a cost-effective manner. However, nutritional care should not simply be viewed as the provision of perioperative or post-injury feeding. Rather, it should be seen as a global strategy of metabolic control, nutritional support and early mobilization, the aim of which is to maximize the rate of recovery and the final nutritional/functional status of the patient.

This chapter will review the basic physiology underlying the metabolic stress response to injury, and detail the clinical administration of artificial nutritional support. In particular, this chapter will describe the guidelines by which surgeons should manage patients of varying pathology and nutritional status. In this way, the reader can develop a strategic understanding of what aspects of clinical care are important, and acquire the appropriate knowledge to manage them.

The Metabolic Stress Response to Surgery and Trauma: The "Ebb and Flow" Model

Any bodily injury, be it operative or accidental, is not only associated with local effects, but is also accompanied by a systemic metabolic response. The main features of this metabolic response are initiated by the immune system, cardiovascular system, sympathetic nervous system, ascending reticular formation and limbic system. However, the metabolic stress response may be further exacerbated by anesthesia, dehydration, starvation (including pre-operative fasting), sepsis, acute medical illness, or even severe psychological stress, and thus any attempt to limit or control these other factors is beneficial to the patient.

In 1930, Sir David Cuthbertson divided the metabolic response to injury into "*ebb*" and "*flow*" phases (Fig. 3.1). The ebb phase begins at the time of injury, and lasts for approximately 24–48 h. It may be attenuated by proper resuscitation, but not completely abolished. The ebb phase is characterized by hypovolemia, decreased basal metabolic rate, reduced cardiac output, hypothermia, and lactic acidosis. The predominant hormones regulating the ebb phase are catecholamines, cortisol and aldosterone (following activation of the renin-angiotensin system). The magnitude of this neuro endocrine response depends on the degree of blood loss and the stimulation of

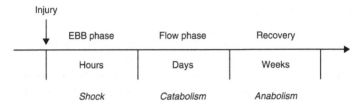

FIGURE 3.1. Phases of the metabolic stress response to injury (After Cuthbertson).

somatic afferent nerves at the site of injury. The main physiological role of the ebb phase is to conserve both circulating volume and energy stores for recovery and repair.

Following resuscitation, the ebb phase evolves into a hypermetabolic flow phase. This phase involves the mobilization of body energy stores for recovery and repair, and the subsequent replacement of lost or damaged tissue. It is characterized by increased basal metabolic rate (hypermetabolism), increased cardiac output, raised body temperature, increased oxygen consumption, and increased gluconeogenesis. The flow phase may be subdivided into an initial catabolic phase, lasting approximately 3–10 days, followed by an anabolic phase, which may last for weeks if extensive recovery and repair are required following serious injury. During the catabolic phase, the increased production of counter-regulatory hormones (including catecholamines, cortisol, insulin and glucagon) and inflammatory cytokines (e.g. interleukin [IL]-1, IL-6 and tumor necrosis factor [TNF]-α) result in significant fat and protein mobilization, leading to significant weight loss and increased urinary nitrogen excretion (Fig. 3.2). The increased production of insulin at this time is associated with significant *insulin resistance* and therefore injured patients often exhibit poor glycemic control. The combination of pronounced or prolonged catabolism, in association with insulin resistance, places patients within this phase at increased risk of complications, particularly infectious and cardiovascular. Obviously the development of complications will further aggravate the neuroendocrine and inflammatory stress responses, thus creating a vicious catabolic cycle.

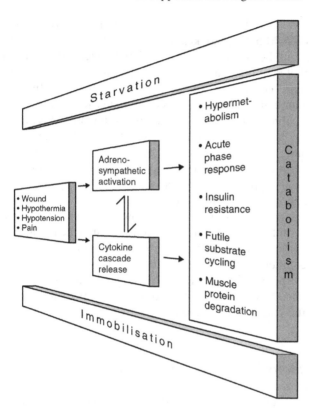

FIGURE 3.2. Key initiators and mechanisms resulting in patient catabolism during the flow phase of the metabolic stress response.

Key Catabolic Elements of the Flow Phase of the Metabolic Stress Response

There are several key elements of the flow phase which determine largely the extent of catabolism and thus govern the nutritional requirements of the surgical patient (Fig. 3.2).

Hypermetabolism

The majority of trauma patients (except possibly those with extensive burns) demonstrate energy expenditures

approximately 15–25% above predicted healthy resting
values (i.e. 1,500–2,500 kcal/day). The predominant cause
appears to be a complex interaction between the central
control of metabolic rate and peripheral energy utilization. In
particular, central thermodysregulation (caused by the
pro-inflammatory cytokine cascade); increased sympathetic
activity; abnormalities in wound circulation (ischemic areas
produce lactate which must be metabolized by the ATP-
consuming hepatic Cori cycle; hyperemic areas cause an
increase in cardiac output); increased protein turnover; and
nutritional support may all increase patient energy expenditure. Theoretically, patient energy expenditure could rise
even higher than observed levels following surgery or trauma,
but several features of standard intensive care (including bed
rest, paralysis, ventilation and external temperature regulation) counteract the hypermetabolic driving forces of the
stress response. Furthermore, the skeletal muscle wasting
experienced by patients with prolonged catabolism actually
limits the volume of metabolically active tissue.

Alterations in Skeletal Muscle Protein Metabolism

Muscle protein is continually synthesized and broken down
each day, with an average turnover rate in humans of 1–2%, and
with a greater amplitude of changes in protein synthesis (±two-
fold) than breakdown (±0.25-fold) during the diurnal cycle.
Under normal circumstances, synthesis equals breakdown and
muscle bulk remains constant. Physiological stimuli that promote
net muscle protein accretion include feeding (especially extracellular amino acid concentration) and exercise. Paradoxically,
during exercise, skeletal muscle protein synthesis is depressed,
but increases again during rest and feeding.

During the catabolic phase of the stress response, muscle
wasting occurs due to an increase in muscle protein degradation (via enzymatic pathways), coupled with a decrease in
muscle protein synthesis. The major site of protein loss is
peripheral skeletal muscle, although nitrogen losses do also

occur in the respiratory muscles (predisposing the patient to hypoventilation and chest infections) and in the gut (reducing gut motility). Cardiac muscle appears to be mostly spared. Under extreme conditions of catabolism (e.g. major sepsis), urinary nitrogen losses can reach 20 g per day; this is equivalent to *600–700 g loss of skeletal muscle per day*.

The predominant mechanism involved in the wasting of skeletal muscle is the ATP-dependent ubiquitin proteasome pathway, although the lysosomal cathepsins and the calcium-calpain pathway play facilitatory and accessory roles.

Clinically, a patient with skeletal muscle wasting will experience asthenia, increased fatigue, reduced functional ability, decreased quality of life, and an increased risk of morbidity and mortality. In critically ill patients, muscle weakness may be further worsened by the development of critical illness myopathy, a multi-factorial condition that is associated with impaired excitation-contraction-coupling at the level of the sarcolemma and the sarcoplasmic reticulum membrane.

Alterations in Hepatic Protein Metabolism: The Acute Phase Protein Response (APPR)

In response to inflammatory conditions, including surgery, trauma, sepsis, cancer or autoimmune conditions, circulating peripheral blood mononuclear cells secrete a range of pro-inflammatory cytokines, including IL-1, IL-6, and tumor necrosis factor (TNF)-α. These cytokines, in particular IL-6, promote the hepatic synthesis of positive acute phase proteins, e.g. fibrinogen and C-reactive protein (CRP). The APPR represents a "double edged sword" for surgical patients as it provides proteins important for recovery and repair, but only at the expense of valuable lean tissue and energy reserves. In contrast to the positive acute phase reactants, the plasma concentrations of other liver export proteins such as albumin (the negative acute phase reactants) fall acutely following injury. However, rather than represent a reduced hepatic synthesis rate, the fall in plasma concentration of negative acute phase reactants is thought, principally, to reflect increased transcapillary escape, secondary to an increase in micro-vascular permeability. Thus, increased hepatic synthesis of positive acute phase reactants is not compensated for by reduced synthesis of negative reactants.

Insulin Resistance

Following surgery or trauma, post-operative hyperglycemia develops as a result of increased glucose production combined with decreased glucose uptake in peripheral tissues. Decreased glucose uptake is a result of insulin resistance that is transiently induced within the stressed patient. Suggested mechanisms for this phenomenon include the action of pro-inflammatory cytokines, and the decreased responsiveness of insulin-regulated glucose transporter proteins. The degree of insulin resistance is proportional to the magnitude of the injurious process. Following routine upper abdominal surgery, insulin resistance may persist for approximately 2 weeks.

Post-operative patients with insulin resistance behave in a similar manner to individuals with Type II diabetes mellitus, and are at increased risk of sepsis, deteriorating renal function, polyneuropathy, and death.

The mainstay management of insulin resistance is intravenous insulin infusion. Insulin infusion may be used in either an *intensive* approach (i.e. sliding scales are manipulated to *normalize* the blood glucose level) or a *conservative* approach (i.e. insulin is administered when the blood glucose level exceeds a defined limit and discontinued when the level falls). Studies of post-operatively ventilated patients in the intensive care unit (ICU) have suggested that maintenance of normal glucose levels using intensive insulin therapy can significantly reduce both morbidity and mortality (Fearon and Luff, 2003). Furthermore, intensive insulin therapy is superior to conservative insulin approaches in reducing morbidity rates. However, the mortality benefit of intensive insulin therapy over a more conservative approach has not been proven conclusively. The observed benefits of insulin therapy are probably simply as a result of maintenance of normoglycemia, but the glycemia-independent actions of insulin may also exert minor, organ-specific effects (e.g. promotion of myocardial systolic function).

The Identification of Patients at Increased Risk of Nutritional Depletion

Ideally, all surgical patients should receive pre-operative nutritional screening. However, formal screening is not performed commonly in clinical practice. A recent study has suggested that only 33% of UK centers performing upper GI cancer resections perform routine pre-operative nutritional screening by dietetic staff (Murphy et al., 2006). However, in the same study, 75% of centers stated that they would commence routinely pre-operative nutritional support if a patient was found to be malnourished on admission. It therefore seems vital that medical staff encourage and are capable of performing basic nutritional assessment, and are also able to identify risk factors that predispose the surgical patient to an increased risk (Table 3.1).

Simple and inexpensive measures of nutritional status that indicate patients are at increased risk include body weight loss >10%, body mass index (BMI) <18 kg/m^2, and the well-recognized, but non-specific risk index of significant hypoalbuminemia (<30 g/l).

An alternative method of assessment is to measure functional status and thus make an indirect judgment regarding

TABLE 3.1. Risk factors associated with nutritional depletion.

- Old age

- Physical inactivity

- Cancer

- Upper gastrointestinal surgery

- Ongoing sepsis

- Impaired oral intake

nutritional status. Subjective assessment of functional status is usually performed using a score of performance status (PS), e.g. Karnofsky performance score (KPS) or the World Health Organisation (WHO) score. These are the most robust treatment risk indices in medical oncology and are easily applied in the pre-operative surgical setting. Objective techniques of functional status assessment involve direct measurements of mobility or muscle power (e.g. hand-grip dynamometry, which is a highly accurate prognostic indicator in surgical patients).

Malnutrition scoring systems are available (e.g. prognostic inflammatory nutritional index [PINI], mini-nutritional assessment [MNA]), but they are not readily used in clinical practice. Furthermore, a variety of strategies have been suggested for screening patients for malnutrition in the community, but it is not clear whether their implementation reduces morbidity or mortality.

The Aim of Nutritional Support in the Surgical Patient

For well-nourished patients, the primary objective of post-operative care is the restoration of normal GI function to allow adequate food intake and rapid recovery. This objective should be carried out within the context of an "enhanced recovery after surgery (ERAS)" protocol or "fast track" surgery program. Within these multimodal codes of surgical practice, strategies are taken to minimize the surgical stress response and to avoid traditional principles of surgical care which have been shown to have no benefit, or are actually detrimental, to the rapid recovery of the patient (Fig. 3.3). In particular, strict attention is paid to pain control, early mobilization and the promotion of GI function (Table 3.2). Furthermore, the patient is well-counseled and encouraged to take an active role in their own post-operative recovery. To date, most ERAS programs have targeted patients undergoing GI (primarily colon) surgery, and have shown that the implementation of modern "stress-fee" surgical practice can minimize deterioration in physiological function and reduce

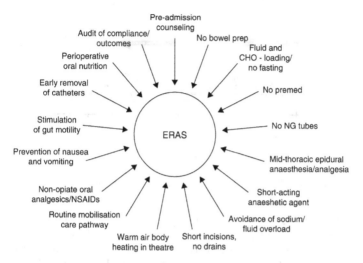

FIGURE 3.3. Key elements of the Enhanced Recovery After Surgery (ERAS) protocol. CHO = carbohydrate; NSAIDs = non-steroidal anti-inflammatory drugs.

TABLE 3.2. Main objectives of the Enhanced Recovery After Surgery (ERAS) protocol.

- Optimize pain relief

- Optimize gut function

- Early mobilization

time to hospital discharge. Indeed, use of an epidural (which allows for dynamic pain control, early mobilization, reduction of post-operative ileus, and blockade of the neuroendocrine stress response) combined with early enteral feeding can result in elective abdominal surgery where the patient remains in positive nitrogen balance with no net losses.

In at-risk malnourished patients, the aim of perioperative nutritional support is to avoid the postoperative complications and increased mortality which are associated with malnutrition (Fig. 3.4). In these individuals, evidence suggests that artificial nutritional support can reduce the length of stay, decrease morbidity, improve quality of life, and

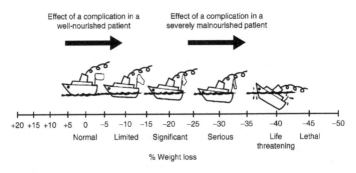

FIGURE 3.4. Effects of weight loss on patient outcome.

consequently limit the cost of health care resources. However, to achieve these goals, one must know when (and how) to administer the relevant nutritional support. In contrast with surgical practice in the 1970s and 1980s, modern "stress-free" anesthesia/perioperative care means that from a strategic viewpoint, even if the patient is *moderately* malnourished, *pre-operative* nutritional support is of limited benefit. Instead, the best management is to proceed with surgery, and once the primary pathology has been dealt with, provide the patient with aggressive *post-operative* nutritional support.

In patients who are *severely* malnourished, it is often prudent to review operative strategy and consider in benign disease whether there are any medical options that could be followed. In severely malnourished patients with malignant disease, consideration should be given to whether the patient has been understaged and if resectional surgery is really the appropriate path to follow (e.g. consider downstaging or stenting).

Nutritional Management of Well-Nourished and Malnourished Surgical Patients

The Well-Nourished Surgical Patient

Patients should be managed within the context of an ERAS protocol, with an emphasis on dynamic pain relief, early mobilization and the restoration of normal GI function.

As well as adhering to the principles of "stress-free" surgery, it is important for the surgeon to have a global strategy to maintain patients' food intake. Key issues are shown in (Fig. 3.3) and include:

- *Avoid routine placement of nasogastric decompression tubes.* Nasogastric tubes are of no proven benefit and prevent restoration of normal food intake.
- *Avoid routine use of bowel preparation except in special circumstances* (e.g. low anterior resection with covering loop ileostomy). If bowel preparation is used, provide the patient with simultaneous low residue oral nutritional supplements.
- *Provide oral fluids up to 2 h prior to operation and consider routine use of oral carbohydrate and fluid loading.* The latter has been proven to reduce post-operative insulin resistance and thus allows the patient to respond to nutritional support more effectively.
- *Use strategies to reduce post-operative ileus.* Routine use of a thoracic epidural blocks reflex sympathetic inhibition of small bowel mobility and is proven to improve gut function postoperatively.
- *Avoid excessive administration of intravenous saline in the intra-operative and post-operative period.* Intravenous saline is proven to cause gut edema, delayed gastric emptying, and worsened patient outcome. Start the patient on oral fluids on the first post-operative day and discontinue the intravenous infusion.
- *Feed the patient early in the post-operative period.* Many surgeons believe that oral feeding cannot be commenced until bowel movements have begun. Furthermore, many others believe that early feeding is associated with increased risks of anastomotic leakage. Neither of these perceptions has been proven on clinical studies. A meta-analysis of controlled trials of early enteral feeding versus nil by mouth after GI surgery concluded that there is no clear advantage to keeping patients nil by mouth after elective GI resection. Early feeding reduced both the risk of any type of infection and the mean length of stay in hospital. However, the risk of vomiting did increase in

patients fed early. Therefore, post-operative feeding should be commenced early with prescription of adequate anti-emetics if required.

The provision of appetizing hospital food and access to sufficient nursing staff to help patients who have difficulty in eating is a key issue in helping patients return to a normal food intake. For patients with an anastomosis in the upper GI tract, ingestion of solid food may have to be delayed for several days (e.g. until contrast studies confirm an intact esophageal anastomosis). In the intervening period, patients can be given post-operative enteral feeding either via a jejunostomy or fine-bore nasoenteral feeding tube. This allows maintenance of nutritional status should the patient develop a post-operative complication that retards normal progression towards oral nutrition (e.g. an anastomotic leak). Upper GI cancer patients are often managed in this way. Following colorectal operations where the GI tract remains functional, solid food can be commenced without adverse effect on the first post-operative day. However, patients may find liquid supplements easier to take in the first instance. Generally, if oral nutrition is not re-established within 5–7 days post-operatively, enteral or parenteral feeding should be considered.

Post-operative energy and protein requirements depend on body composition, clinical status and mobility. However, an estimation of requirements is 30 kcal/kg/day and 1 g protein/kg/day for the average patient. Few patients require more than 2,200 kcal/day. Additional calories are unlikely to be used effectively and may constitute a metabolic stress.

The Moderately/Severely Malnourished Surgical Patient

Studies suggest that approximately 20–40% of surgical patients may already be malnourished on admission to hospital. Following surgery, these patients have a higher risk of complications, prolonged hospital stay, delayed recovery, and ultimately, increased mortality. The key issue in managing severely malnourished patients is that plans must always be in place to progress their nutritional status back up towards normality. If severely malnourished patients develop complications which inhibit nutritional support (e.g. abdominal sepsis from an anastomotic leak), their nutritional/metabolic problems can suddenly become major determinants of outcome (see Fig. 3.4).

Moderate or severely malnourished patients (e.g. weight loss >15%, BMI <18 kg/m^2, albumin <30g/l) should be identified by pre-operative nutritional screening and should then be referred to the unit dietician or dedicated nutrition team for consideration of not only perioperative, but also postdischarge, artificial nutritional support. This is because patients who are malnourished at the time of GI surgery can demonstrate evidence of deteriorating nutritional status for up to 2 months or more following hospital discharge. In these patients, the provision of nutritional advice and routine oral nutritional supplements (ONS) in the immediate post-operative period and ensuing 2 months has been shown to promote a more rapid recovery of nutritional status, physical function and quality of life. In contrast, the evidence supporting the short term routine use of ONS in patients who have a normal nutritional status is not clear.

Some patients may not tolerate an adequate intake of ONS in the post-operative period. Therefore, placement of a feeding jejunostomy at the time of surgery in malnourished patients at risk of complications is always a good pre-emptive maneuver. A non-functioning GI tract is an early indication to use total parenteral nutrition (TPN), in order to provide bedrock for progress and the gradual introduction of enteral feeding. Once enteral feeding is well tolerated, TPN can be withdrawn.

Despite the evident benefits of *post-operative* nutritional support, there is no clear proof that malnourished patients requiring surgery (e.g. Crohn's disease) benefit from prolonged *pre-operative* artificial nutritional support. Such patients are best treated by surgical correction of their pathology followed by intensive nutritional support in the post-operative period. In patients who are malnourished, it is often wise to reassess

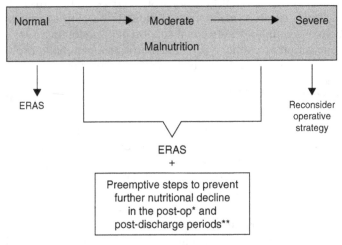

Strategy for nutritional management of
patients undergoing major surgery

FIGURE 3.5. Strategies for the nutritional management of well-nourished, moderately malnourished and severely malnourished patients in the post-operative period. ERAS = Enhanced Recovery After Surgery; EN = enteral nutrition; TPN = total parenteral nutrition.

the necessity and appropriateness of surgery and consider any non-operative medical or palliative options.

Strategies for the nutritional management of well-nourished, moderately malnourished and severely malnourished patients in the post-operative period are summarized in Fig. 3.5.

The Surgical Patient with Post-Operative Complications

Surgery will induce a catabolic state within the patient, placing that individual at increased risk of complications.

The development of post-operative complications will prolong or re-initiate the neuroendocrine and inflammatory stress responses, thus creating a vicious catabolic cycle, and elevating significantly protein and energy requirements. It is therefore vital that these patients receive adequate nutritional support.

The Practicalities of Artificial Nutritional Support

Although artificial nutritional support can be of undoubted benefit, it can also be associated with major complications. Therefore, nutritional support should be monitored closely and regularly (Table 3.3). The measurements and frequency of monitoring depend on the individual patient, the route and the stage of feeding. Daily monitoring should be carried out in unstable patients or patients who have recently started nutritional support. A co-ordinated multidisciplinary team approach can reduce the incidence of complications and improve patients' overall quality of life. The choice of which

TABLE 3.3. Methods to monitor surgical patients who are receiving artificial nutritional support.

Status	Test	Frequency
Biochemistry	Electrolytes	Twice weekly
	Urea	
	Blood glucose	
	Liver function tests	
	Urinalysis	
Fluid balance	Fluid charts	Daily
	Weight	Once weekly
Nutritional status	Weight	Once weekly
	Nitrogen balance	
Nutritional intake	Nursing records	Daily
	Food and fluid charts	

form of support is appropriate to the individual patient will depend on patient disease status and the perceived risk of associated complications.

Oral Nutritional Supplements (ONS)

Provision of post-operative ONS containing 1.5 kcal/ml and 0.06 g/ml of protein have been shown to improve nutritional status, quality of life, and morbidity rate in malnourished patients undergoing GI surgery.

Enteral Nutrition (EN)

EN uses the physiological route of nutrient intake, is cheaper and generally safer, and should be the preferred method of nutritional support in the presence of a functioning GI tract. Most surgical patients can tolerate a standard whole protein feed (1 kcal/ml). A peptide or elemental formula can be considered in patients with significant malabsorption. Patients are generally commenced on 30–50 ml/h, increasing within 24–48 h as gastric aspirates fall and tolerance improves, until prescribed targets are reached.

If supplementation of an inadequate oral intake is required, then overnight feeding for 8–12 h may be sufficient and allows the patient to be mobile during the day. A pump should be used to control the rate of feed delivery, avoiding the abdominal cramps and bloating associated with bolus feeding.

EN can be administered via several different routes:

Nasogastric Feeding: The most appropriate route of enteral tube feeding for patients who require short-term support (e.g. less than 4 weeks) is via a fine-bore nasogastric (NG) tube.

Gastrostomy: Gastrostomy (endoscopic, radiological or surgical) should be reserved for mid- to long-term feeding. It is more comfortable than NG feeding and has a lower risk of tube misplacement or blockage. Major indications include neurological disorders and head and neck cancer. Contra-indications include sepsis, ascites and clotting disorders.

Jejunostomy: Tubes may be placed surgically or endoscopically. The most common indication is following major upper GI surgery. The jejunostomy is sited at the time of surgery and can be used for feeding within 12 h of surgery.

Parenteral Nutrition

Peripheral intravenous feeding (e.g. via a cannula) should only be used in the short-term. Central venous feeding, via either a peripherally-inserted central catheter (PICC line) or a catheter in a central vein, is the preferred route. A dedicated central venous feeding line minimizes infective complications. However, in suitable circumstances a triple lumen central line inserted under aseptic conditions and with a dedicated port for TPN can be used. Following insertion of a central venous line into the internal jugular or subclavian veins, a chest x-ray must be taken to exclude a pneumothorax and confirm the position of the catheter tip at or near the junction of the superior vena cava with the right atrium. Furthermore, care should be taken during line insertion to exclude arterial puncture and the risk of bleeding.

Mixtures of nutrients are usually combined in a single bag. Many pharmacies now use three or four standard regimens. The solutions contain fixed amounts of energy and nitrogen, and typically provide 1,800–2,400 kcals (50% glucose, 50% lipid) and 10–14 g nitrogen. The amount of electrolytes, vitamins and trace elements can be varied. In general, standard regimens are simpler, safer and cheaper than those prepared individually. However, nutritional requirements should always be determined in consultation with a dietician.

Historically, TPN has been associated with an increased risk of patient infection. These infections may have been the result of infected intravenous access, or a result of carbohydrate overloading and subsequent hyperglycemia. However, in many of these studies, the TPN solutions in question lacked glutamine. The subsequent addition of glutamine or glutamine dipeptides to standard TPN in order to enhance immune function has the potential to improve outcome.

TPN is of benefit in the treatment of severely malnourished patients and post-operative patients with GI complications. However, the routine use of post operative TPN is not beneficial in patients capable of eating within 5–7 days of an operation.

Daily biochemical monitoring must be undertaken when initially re-feeding the chronically severely malnourished patient because of the dangers of hypocalcemia and hypophosphatemia.

Immunonutrition

Feeds which contain immune-enhancing agents (e.g. arginine, branched chain amino acids, omega-3 fatty acids, dietary nucleotides) may be given pre-operatively and/or post-operatively. It has been suggested that these compound feeds may be particularly advantageous in the management of patients with cancer and multiple injuries, but evidence for both efficacy and cost-effectiveness is currently unclear. A meta-analysis has demonstrated that EN supplemented with immunomodulatory nutrients results in significant reduction in the risk of developing infectious complications but has no effect on mortality. Furthermore, other studies have suggested that some immunomodulatory formations are associated with an increased risk of mortality in critically ill patients.

Conclusion

Nutritional support should be considered as a global strategy of reducing nutritional depletion and maximizing patient recovery. The correct use of nutritional support can inhibit the deleterious effects of the metabolic stress response on patient nutrition; can accelerate recovery in elective surgical patients; and can be life-saving in malnourished patients, especially those who develop post-operative major complications.

Further studies are required to optimize both the composition of current feeds and their application.

Selected Readings

Beattie AH, Prach AT, Baxter JP, Pennington CR (2000) A randomised controlled trial evaluating the use of enteral nutritional supplements postoperatively in malnourished surgical patients. Gut 46:813–818

Fearon KC, Luff R (2003) The nutritional management of surgical patients: enhanced recovery after surgery. Proc Nutr Soc 62:807–811

Fearon KC, Ljungqvist Von O, Meyenfeldt M, et al. (2005) Enhanced recovery after surgery: a consensus review of clinical care for patients undergoing colonic resection. Clin Nutr 24:466–477

Ljungqvist O, Fearon KC, Little RA (2005) Nutrition in surgery and trauma. In: Gibney MJ, Marinos E, Ljungqvist O, Dowsett J (eds) Clinical nutrition. Blackwell Science, Oxford, pp. 312–324

Murphy PM, Modi P, Rahamim J, et al. (2006) An investigation into the current perioperative nutritional management of oesophageal carcinoma patients in major carcinoma centers in England. Ann R Coll Surg Engl 88:358–362

Nygren J, Hausel J, Kehlet H, et al. (2005) A comparison in five European Centres of case mix, clinical management and outcomes following either conventional or fast-track perioperative care in colorectal surgery. Clin Nutr 24:455–461

O'Riordain MG, Falconer JS, Maingay J, et al. (1999) Peripheral blood cells from weight-losing cancer patients control the hepatic acute phase response by a primarily interleukin-6 dependent mechanism. Int J Oncol 15:823–827

O'Riordain MG, Fearon KC, Ross JA, et al. (1994) Glutamine supplemented total parenteral nutrition enhances T lymphocyte response in surgical patients undergoing colorectal resection. Ann Surg 220:212–221

Tambyraja AL, Sengupta F, MacGregor AB, et al. (2004) Patterns and clinical outcomes associated with routine intravenous sodium and fluid administration after colorectal resection. World J Surg 28:1046–1051

Van den Berghe G, Wouters P, Weekers F, et al. (2001) Intensive insulin therapy in the critically ill patients. N Engl J Med 345:1359–1367

Van den Berghe G, Wilmer A, Hermans G, et al. (2006) Intensive insulin therapy in the medical ICU. N Engl J Med 354:449–461

4
Abnormal Bleeding and Coagulopathies

Randy J. Woods and Mary C. McCarthy

Pearls and Pitfalls

- Resuscitation of the bleeding patient with isotonic saline solutions will rapidly dilute and deplete the clotting system.
- In patients who respond to fluids but appear to have continued moderate blood loss, angiography and embolization may be of value in stopping continued bleeding if deemed not to be surgically controllable.
- Prevention and correction of acidosis and hypothermia is essential for the optimal function of platelets and clotting factors.
- In the stable patient, using coagulation studies to guide component replacement is effective.
- However, in the face of massive hemorrhage, awaiting coagulation studies will prolong the duration of shock and coagulopathy.
- It is vital to anticipate the need for blood products. Patients arriving with a significant base deficit or ongoing hemorrhage will require FFP, platelets, and/or cryoprecipitate.
- Blood products and the best ICU care will not take the place of adequate surgical control of hemorrhage.
- Damage control procedures in the injured patient should be performed prior to the onset of coagulopathy. High-risk patients have an injury severity score >25, pH < 7.3, T < 35°C, systolic blood pressure <90 mmHg, base deficit >6, and lactate >4 mmol/l.

K.I. Bland et al. (eds.), *General Principles of Surgery*,
DOI 10.1007/978-1-84996-381-7_4,
© Springer-Verlag London Limited 2011

Recent advances in the care of the bleeding surgical patient have resulted in a significant decrease in the morbidity and mortality of major injuries. Concepts such as "damage control surgery," improved blood banking techniques, a better understanding of component therapy, and increased awareness of the impact of the "lethal triad" (hypothermia, acidosis, and coagulopathy) have enabled surgeons to successfully control severe hemorrhage. Understanding the physiology of the coagulation system, the clinical presentation of inherited and acquired coagulopathies, and appropriate treatment options enable the surgeon to provide optimal care for the bleeding patient.

Physiology of the Coagulation System

The traditional intrinsic and extrinsic model of the coagulation cascade has been replaced by the cell-based model, in which platelets, endothelium, and inflammatory cells interact in the production of thrombus and mature clot. Hemostasis is a three-stage process which includes: (1) primary hemostasis (initiation) occurs when activated platelets stimulated by the presence of tissue factor (TF) form a plug within minutes; (2) secondary hemostasis (amplification) occurs when the immature platelet plug is reinforced with fibrin strands; and (3) fibrinolysis, dissolves the clot after the vascular endothelium has been repaired, which occurs over a period of days.

In the current understanding of hemostasis, cells such as those of the vascular endothelium have acquired a larger role. Breakdown of the endothelial layer exposes collagen and TF to circulating platelets and leukocytes, causing the platelets to adhere and plug the disrupted vessel. Once activated, the platelets act as a catalyst for secondary hemostasis. Amplification occurs when the tissue factor stimulated cell membranes bind Factor VII and act as a catalyst for the large-scale production of thrombin. The activated platelets express adhesion molecules that interact with leukocytes causing activation and amplification of processes involving cytokines and cofactors. This crossover into the inflammatory system helps to explain the activation of both inflammation and coagulation in septic and bleeding patients. In systemic immune response syndrome (SIRS), circulating cytokines stimulate coagulation, causing the development of microemboli and progressing to multiple system organ failure (MSOF). This observation helps to explain how manipulating the coagulation system can result in improvement in organ failure due to SIRS or sepsis.

Clinical Presentation of Coagulopathies

Inherited Coagulopathies

In preparing for elective surgery or evaluating a trauma patient, a thorough history and physical exam should be performed. Questions about prior mucosal bleeding tendencies, easy bruising, or previous episodes of hemarthrosis have taken the place of routine coagulation testing. Further evaluation for bleeding dyscrasias should be prompted by positive responses to the pertinent review of systems or family history. In general, mucosal bleeding and subcutaneous bleeding are indicative of platelet dysfunction. Deep muscle bleeding or hemarthrosis is typical of factor deficiencies. The initial evaluation should consist of a complete blood count (CBC) assessing for anemia and a quantitative platelet count, protime (PT), activated partial thromboplastin time (aPTT), and a platelet function study.

Inherited platelet membrane receptor defects are not uncommon, with von Willebrand disease (vWD) being the most common deficiency. Occasionally the aPTT will be slightly elevated. It is important to identify the correct subtype of vWD so that proper treatment can be initiated.

Inherited factor deficiencies are also common, with the hemophilias being the most prevalent. Patients with hemophilia will have histories of hemarthrosis, spontaneous muscle hematomas, and gastrointestinal bleeding. Inherited deficiencies of factor VIII (hemophilia A) and factor IX (hemophilia B) require factor replacement and monitoring of treatment factor levels in the cases of trauma or surgery. In general, with the proper evaluation and perioperative factor replacement, elective and even acute surgical emergencies can be safely managed in patients with hemophilia.

Acquired Coagulopathies

Patients are now living longer and receiving chronic treatment for atrial fibrillation, carotid artery atherosclerosis, and valvular disease. Treatment may include drugs that interfere with the normal clotting cascade. Therefore, acquired coagulopathies are increasingly common. Active and otherwise healthy patients are receiving medications such as aspirin, warfarin, ibuprofen and other nonsteroidal anti-inflammatory drugs (NSAIDs), clopidogrel, and ticlopidine. Generally these medications have a good risk:benefit ratio. However, when a patient simply falls from the standing position, the risk of intracranial hemorrhage and death increases if rapid reversal of these agents is not initiated promptly.

Acquired platelet abnormalities are common and can be either qualitative (aspirin or clopidogrel therapy) or quantitative (myelodysplastic disorder). Platelet function studies can be helpful when a patient's medication history is unknown, for example, when they arrive in the emergency department with an intracranial hemorrhage after a fall at home. However, recent personal experience has demonstrated that a normal platelet function test does not guarantee that coagulation will proceed normally.

Hemodilutional Coagulopathy

Hemodilutional coagulopathy develops in patients with ongoing hemorrhage. If the coagulopathy is not treated promptly, the patient will deteriorate to irreversible shock.

This may be related to a cellular change such as apoptosis or exhaustion of physiologic reserves. The factors of the lethal triad – hypothermia, acidosis and coagulopathy – may contribute to this resistant shock state. Resuscitation of the bleeding patient with isotonic saline solutions will rapidly dilute the components of the clotting system. Hemorrhage up to one blood volume and replacement with packed red blood cells (PRBC) alone will result in a 70% decrease in the coagulation factors. The remaining coagulation factors are usually sufficient to prevent a bleeding diathesis (Ingerslev and Hvid, 2006). However, acidosis and hypothermia are frequently seen in patients with traumatic shock and compound the problem. Ischemia-reperfusion injury to the endothelium after delayed or inadequate volume resuscitation or a soft tissue crush injury from blunt trauma can also result in significant consumption of factors. Early transfusion of packed red blood cells alone will result in depletion of coagulation factors and other components of successful clotting. One must keep in mind that the patient is bleeding more than just red blood cells. Component therapy using banked RBCs has replaced the use of fresh whole blood. Therefore the other coagulation elements must also be replaced.

In trauma patients, exsanguination is one of the leading causes of death (Lavoie et al., 2004). Ongoing hemorrhage and increased utilization of factors and other elements of the clotting cascade compound this problem. Early initiation of packed red blood cells and transfusion of fresh frozen plasma (FFP) or thawed plasma, cryoprecipitate, and platelets are needed to reverse the coagulopathy in actively bleeding patients. FFP contains all the essential clotting factors, including fibrinogen, although the fibrinogen level in FFP is less than that in cryoprecipitate. It is important to anticipate the use of FFP because it requires 30 min to thaw. The clotting factors in FFP are crucial for the conversion of fibrinogen to fibrin for clot formation. In the massively bleeding patient, fibrinogen will be one of the first factors to be depleted, and administration of cryoprecipitate may also be required. Cryoprecipitate is also stored frozen, but due to its smaller volume, can be available in 10–20 min.

Recombinant factor VIIa (rFVIIa) is a recent addition to the armamentarium to correct coagulopathy. Recombinant FVIIa is approved in the management of patients with hemophilia A who have demonstrated antibodies to factor VIII. Recombinant FVIIa does not have an approved indication for use in trauma surgical patients, although there have been studies showing benefit. There is also evidence that the use of rFVIIa improves coagulation studies and reduces the amount of blood loss. Exogenous factor VII binds to circulating tissue factor (TF) at the site of the endothelial injury. Factor VII then activates factors IX and X, which ultimately results in a burst of thrombin generation.

Disseminated Intravascular Coagulation

Disseminated intravascular coagulation (DIC) is a consequence of an underlying disease and not a process itself (see Table 4.1). DIC should be thought of as systemic endothelial dysfunction in which the usually anticoagulant endothelium becomes a stimulus for a hypercoagulable state. Optimal results in the treatment of DIC are achieved following an

TABLE 4.1. Etiologies of DIC.

Sepsis (gram-negative infection)
Traumatic shock
Delayed resuscitation in shock
Ischemic or necrotic tissue
Abscess
Cancers (acute leukemia and metastatic prostatic carcinomas)
Severe traumatic brain injury
Severe thermal injury
Fat embolism
Complicated birth
Transfusion reaction

aggressive search for its etiology and treatment. DIC stems from tissue factor (TF) expression on a multitude of cell surfaces. One possible source of TF is endothelial injury due to sepsis. As stated previously, the TF causes activation of factors VII and IX, which ultimately leads to thrombin generation. Unlike normal clotting events, the TF in DIC is not localized to the injured site, thereby causing a local process to become systemic. This uncontrolled activation of factors VII and IX causes activation of the clotting process at all levels. If the consumption of coagulation factors outpaces production, then uncompensated DIC occurs. The patient then becomes hypocoagulable and bleeding occurs. If the underlying cause of DIC is untreated, clotting factors will be consumed and fibrin split products (degradation products from the fibrinolytic process) will increase. Platelet count and fibrinogen levels decrease, while PT/INR, aPTT, and D-dimer levels increase. Mortality in septic patients with DIC is double that of patients without DIC. As DIC progresses, fibrin microemboli occlude the microvasculature of end organs, resulting in local hypoperfusion and eventually MSOF.

The diagnosis of DIC depends on whether the patient is in a hypercoagulable state (consumption of clotting products matched by production) or hypocoagulable state (consumption outpaces the production). Signs of thrombosis include mental status changes, tissue ischemia (seen in the fingertips of the hand with a radial arterial line), renal insufficiency, respiratory failure, and gastrointestinal ulceration. Classic signs in the hypocoagulable state include intracranial bleeding, skin petechia and ecchymosis, mucosal bleeding, hematuria, and gastrointestinal bleeding. Retroperitoneal bleeding may be manifest by a falling hematocrit.

The treatment of DIC begins with resuscitation and rapid transfusion of PRBC, if indicated. Persistent shock will result in refractory DIC with increased mortality; prompt resuscitation is vital. In patients experiencing major thrombotic events (limb-threatening ischemia) heparin, or low molecular weight heparin may be beneficial. However, correcting the underlying etiology of the DIC is paramount to successful recovery of the patient. Abnormal PT/INR should be corrected with FFP, severe thrombocytopenia (platelet count <50,000/mm^3) with platelet transfusions, and fibrinogen levels replenished to above 100 mg/dl with cryoprecipitate.

In the setting of sepsis-associated DIC with organ system dysfunction, activated protein C may be of benefit. In patients with Acute Physiology and Chronic Health Evaluation (APACHE) II Scores greater than 25, activated protein C shows promise in reversing organ dysfunction with an acceptable risk of bleeding.

Treatment

The initial treatment of the bleeding patient will depend upon the etiology of hemorrhage. Patients with inherited coagulopathies will need initial factor replacement and maintenance of therapeutic levels. A hematology consult may be helpful in management. However, patients who are bleeding due to prolonged or inadequate resuscitation from shock, massive transfusion, or an acquired coagulopathy need to be addressed differently.

First, the surgeon should ensure that blood loss is not the result of inadequate surgical control. When a patient's blood pressure is low and a damage control procedure is performed, bleeding may be controlled temporarily. With continued resuscitation, rewarming, and normalization of the blood pressure, bleeding that was initially controlled may resume. A return to the operating room may be needed to re-explore the operative field. Blood products and rigorous intensive care will not take the place of adequate surgical control of significant bleeding. In patients who respond to fluids but appear to have continued moderate blood loss, angiography and embolization may be valuable. This is especially true if the initial exploration did not reveal the bleeding source, or if bleeding is deep within the liver parenchyma, in the retroperitoneum, or along the pelvic sidewall from a complex pelvic fracture.

Laboratory studies such as PT/INR, aPTT, qualitative and quantitative platelet studies can be used to direct component replacement. Diffuse oozing in the operative site is an indicator of hypothermia and/or a platelet defect. Bloody return from operative drains can be caused by many factors. In a stable patient, using coagulation studies to guide component replacement is effective. However, in the face of massive hemorrhage, awaiting coagulation studies will prolong the duration of the coagulation abnormality. This results in continued blood loss, hypoperfusion, and further endothelial injury, with consequent DIC. In complex situations, thromboelastography (TEG) allows more rapid point-of-care testing for platelet function, enzyme activity, and fibrinolysis. Evaluating fibrinolysis may help in determining mild cases of DIC and prompt an earlier evaluation for an etiology.

Intraoperatively, packing the site of injury to control bleeding and truncating the procedure to concentrate on control of hypothermia and coagulopathy is necessary. Return to the operating room in 24–72 h for completion of the surgical procedure should be planned. In the majority of patients, aggressive rewarming and resuscitation is needed. Initially factor repletion is empiric, and later coagulation studies are used as a guide. Formulas for component replacement based on number of PRBC transfused can be wasteful (Ingerslev and Hvid, 2006). However, transfusion formulas are useful triggers to remind providers that PRBC are devoid of platelets or clotting factors. Ongoing clinical evidence of bleeding or laboratory assessment should guide further transfusion of blood products.

After control of hemorrhage and enteric spill in a damage control procedure, what remains in the short-term is aggressive correction of an acquired coagulopathy. In many institutions, the short trip from the OR to the ICU is enough to result in a further delay in resuscitation. It may be helpful to delay transfer to the ICU and continue resuscitation in the OR. Rapid infusion devices that deliver 1–2 l/min of warmed blood and blood products can quickly replace needed factors. Care must be taken not to overload the patient, but this time spent before transfer can be lifesaving in the appropriate patient. Although surgical blood salvage (cell saver) should be used whenever possible, the recycled red blood cells will be critically low in essential clotting factors and platelets. Therefore, salvaged blood used in resuscitation will require FFP, platelets, and at times, cryoprecipitate to be administered in conjunction with recycled washed red blood cells.

Mentioned earlier, rFVIIa has been shown to reduce hemorrhage in trauma patients. More work needs to be done refining the optimal patient population, appropriate timing of the product, and the accompanying risks and complications. There is no consensus on the dosage of rFVIIa in trauma patients or those with intracranial hemorrhage. A randomized trial in trauma has recently been completed in the United States. Hypothermia and acidosis should be corrected prior to the administration of rFVIIa (Meng et al., 2003). The drug is very expensive, and therefore, most trauma centers have developed protocols for its use (see Table 4.2).

Although often difficult, preventing hypothermia and acidosis is the best strategy to minimize coagulopathy. Prompt resuscitation of patients reduces endothelial injury and decreases MSOF, infectious complications, and death. There are many tools at the surgeon's disposal to facilitate these goals. The surgeon should become familiar with the concepts reviewed here and be ready to initiate treatment promptly.

TABLE 4.2. Protocol for use of activated recombinant factor Vii (rFVIIa).

Before using rFVIIa in the coagulopathic patient address

- Serum pH > 7.2

- Temperature > 35°C

- Platelet count > 50,000 mm^3

- Fibrinogen > 100 mg/dl

Initial dose of 100 mcg/kg body weight (may need to be repeated)

Selected Readings

Dutton RP, McCunn M, Hyder M, et al. (2004) Factor VIIa for correction of traumatic coagulopathy. J Trauma 57:709–718; discussion 718

Erber WN, Perry DJ (2006) Plasma and plasma products in the treatment of massive haemorrhage. Best Pract Res Clin Haematol 19:97–112

Ingerslev J, Hvid I (2006) Surgery in hemophilia. the general view: patient selection, timing, and preoperative assessment. Semin Hematol 43:S23–S26

Lavoie A, Ratte S, Clas D, et al. (2004) Preinjury warfarin use among elderly patients with closed head injuries in a trauma center. J Trauma 56:802–807

MacLeod JB, Lynn M, McKenney MG, et al. (2003) Early coagulopathy predicts mortality in trauma. J Trauma 55:39–44

5
Blood Transfusion and Alternative Therapies

Henry M. Cryer

Pearls and Pitfalls

- Blood transfusion is substantially overutilized and has significant associated risk, including: transfusion reactions, transmission of blood borne pathogens, and immune suppression.
- The accepted transfusion "trigger" in euvolemic patients is 7 gm/dl for healthy individuals and 8–9 gm/dl for patients with co-morbidities associated with decreased cardiopulmonary reserve.
- Blood transfusion is an independent predictor of MOF, SIRS, increased infection, and mortality in patients with severe injuries and undergoing complex surgical procedures.
- Transfusion of only the amount of blood that maximizes immediate survival and minimizes late inflammatory complications is the goal of resuscitation.
- Trauma patients and other patients in hemorrhagic shock should be transfused based upon blood pressure, pulse, and other measurements of decreased perfusion rather than relying upon laboratory values.
- "The triad of death" including bleeding, hypothermia, and acidosis, leads to the "bloody vicious cycle" of hemorrhage, resuscitation, hemodilution, coagulopathy, and continued bleeding.

K.I. Bland et al. (eds.), *General Principles of Surgery*,
DOI 10.1007/978-1-84996-381-7_5,
© Springer-Verlag London Limited 2011

- "Damage control" strategies that control immediately life-threatening injuries and hemorrhage and wait until normal physiology has been restored in the ICU prior to definitive repair of injuries have been adopted to avoid the "bloody vicious cycle".
- Massive blood loss requires rapid decisions.
- Massive transfusion must be anticipated and massive transfusion protocols instituted prior to the development of coagulopathy.
- One proposed massive transfusion protocol utilizes a 1:1:1 ratio of PRBC, FFP and platelets.
- Alternate each unit of blood with FFP and then give 16-pack of platelets after each 6 units of blood.

Introduction

Blood transfusion is integral to the success of advanced surgical procedures on the heart, transplantation, joint replacement, major cancer resections, and major injury. When patients lose blood either from injury or an operation, blood transfusion has the obvious benefit of restoring oxygen carrying capacity to maintain the metabolic demands of organs and tissues. On the other hand, there are definite risks and consequences of the infusion of blood products including transfusion reaction, transmission of blood borne pathogens, and immune suppression. As with any therapy, it is important to establish a risk-benefit profile for the various clinical situations in which blood transfusion is considered during the care of surgical patients.

Potential Benefits of Blood Transfusion

It is obvious that blood loss leads to lack of oxygen carrying capacity, decreased tissue perfusion, and ultimately organ failure and death if allowed to proceed below a critical threshold. This threshold is different depending on the circumstances in which bleeding occurs. Sudden loss of blood as occurs after major vascular injury can result in profound hemorrhagic shock and sudden death if control of bleeding and volume restoration do not occur rapidly. On the other hand, with gradual loss of blood as usually occurs during elective surgical operations, continuous intravascular volume repletion leads to euvolemic anemia rather than profound hemorrhagic shock. Under conditions of euvolemic anemia, it has been established that the lower threshold for hemoglobin concentration, below which organ function cannot be maintained, is in the neighborhood of 5–6 g/dl. This threshold may be somewhat higher in patients that have underlying decreases in physiologic reserve such as patients with coronary artery disease, or patients with chronic obstructive pulmonary disease. Signs and symptoms of decreased perfusion are rather subtle at a hemoglobin level of 5 g/dl, where hemodynamics are maintained, but decreases in mentation occur. By the time the hemoglobin reaches approximately 3 g/dl patients become comatose and begin to have ST segment changes indicative of impending myocardial infarction. Given these findings, the currently accepted blood transfusion trigger is a hemoglobin level of 7 g/dl in an otherwise euvolemic patient with relatively normal health. Patients with decreased physiologic reserve usually have a transfusion trigger somewhat higher at the 8–9 g/dl range. Patients undergoing acute blood loss should be transfused if active hemorrhage is not controlled and there is evidence of hypovolemia, such as decreased blood pressure and tachycardia.

Consequences of Blood Transfusion

The obvious benefit of blood transfusion is to improve oxygen carrying capacity and restore tissue perfusion with oxygen and nutrients. Counterbalancing these potential benefits are a number of deleterious consequences of blood transfusion. Immediate risks include allergic, febrile, and hemolytic transfusion reactions, acute pulmonary edema, and anaphylaxis. Delayed risks include transmission of Human Immunodeficiency Virus

TABLE 5.1. Estimated risk of transfusion
(Modified from Madjidpour, et al. 2005).

HIV	1:1.5M–1:4.7M
HBV	1:31K–1:205K
HCV	1:2M–1:3M
Bacterial sepsis	1:30K–1:140K
Malaria	1:4M
Acute hemolysis	1:13K
Delayed hemolysis	1:9K
TRALI	1:4K–1:500K
Mistransfusion	1:14K–1:18K

(HIV), Hepatitis C Virus (HCV), Hepatitis B Virus (HBV) and other as yet poorly characterized or undiscovered pathogens. The blood supply is regulated differently in different countries, so there is some variability in the risks of these complications. Estimates for Western countries are listed in Table 5.1. Over 10,000,000 units of packed red blood cells are transfused annually in the United States with only 30–40 deaths nationwide thought to be caused by these transfusions. This equates to roughly 1 death per 300,000 transfusions. It is important to remember this figure when considering alternatives to blood transfusion. The most dangerous complication is a major hemolytic reaction caused by ABO incompatibility resulting in the lysis of donor RBCs. The clinical presentation of ABO incompatibility is immediate occurring within minutes of the initiation of the blood transfusion. The patient becomes tachypneic, hypotensive and extremely anxious. There may be high fever, evidence of diffuse microvascular bleeding, the development of renal failure, disseminated intravascular coagulation (DIC) and death. This reaction usually results from a clerical error and occurs very rarely at a rate approximately 1 per 700,000 units of blood transfused. Treatment is to stop the transfusion immediately and support the circulation with intravenous fluids, mechanical ventilation and supportive care. Non-hemolytic febrile and other allergic reactions also occur with varying severity ranging from mild urticaria to severe lymphangioedema and acute lung injury (TRALI).

In trauma patients, blood transfusion has been identified as an independent predictor of multiple organ failure (MOF), systemic inflammatory response syndrome (SIRS), increased infection, and increased mortality. Furthermore, the cumulative risk appears to be linearly correlated with the number of units transfused, the length of storage time, and the presence of donor leucocytes. Whether blood transfusion is simply a surrogate measure of severity of hemorrhagic shock or it is the blood transfusion itself which leads to these problems has been difficult to ascertain. However, the distinction is somewhat moot, since the problem requiring multiple blood transfusions is always present when blood transfusion occurs. It is clear that transfusion of six or more units of blood during the first 24 hours (h) after injury is associated with a profound pro-inflammatory response and increased risk for MOF, infection and immune suppression. While there is also evidence that transfusion of even one unit of blood can increase the risk of these complications, the magnitude of the effect is less clear.

Immunosuppression is also a consequence of allogeneic blood transfusion and in some studies is associated with increased risk of cancer recurrence after potentially curative surgery, as well as increased frequency of postoperative bacterial infection. Furthermore, this infection risk is higher in patients requiring blood transfusion with traumatic injury compared to those receiving transfusion during or after elective surgery. While the mechanism is still unclear, increased storage time of blood has been associated with the generation of inflammatory mediators and neutrophil activation. Leukoreduction of banked blood has the theoretic benefit of avoiding the immune effects associated with white blood cells and is now uniformly practiced in many European countries. Additionally, free hemoglobin, which occurs as a result of hemolysis of old red blood cells, increases significantly as blood storage time increases. This free hemoglobin can bind to nitric oxide and interfere with regulation of microvascular tone, leading to a mismatch of supply and demand in the microcirculation.

Guidelines for Blood Transfusion

Given the significant risk of allogenic blood transfusion, a risk-benefit analysis must be undertaken prior to the transfusion of blood. The American Society of Anesthesia has published a consensus practice guideline for peri-operative blood transfusion and adjuvant therapies and similar guidelines have been published in Europe. These guidelines focus on the peri-operative management of patients undergoing surgery or other invasive procedures in which significant blood loss occurs or is expected.

Preoperative Decisions Regarding Blood Transfusion

Pre-operative evaluation should include a review of prior medical records, a physical examination, an interview of the patient or family to identify risk factors, and a laboratory evaluation to include at least a hemoglobin level, hematocrit and coagulation profile. If patients have increased potential for organ ischemia, such as cardiorespiratory disease, this may influence the ultimate transfusion trigger. Patients taking anticoagulation medications such as clopidogrel, coumadin or aspirin may require increased transfusion of blood and non-red blood cell components such as fresh frozen plasma and platelets. Additionally, a pre-operative evaluation should include checking for the presence of congenital or acquired blood disorders, the use of vitamins or herbal supplements that may affect coagulation, (Table 5.2) and previous exposure to drugs such as aprotinin that may cause an allergic reaction upon repeated exposure.

TABLE 5.2. Vitamins and herbal supplements that may affect blood loss (Blajchman, 2006).

Herbal supplements that decrease platelet aggregation
Bilberry
Bromelain
Dong quoi
Feverfew
Fish oil
Flax seed oil
Garlic
Ginger
Gingko biloba
Grape seed extract
Saw palmetto
Herbs that inhibit clotting
Chamomile
Dandelion root
Dong quoi
Horse chestnut
Vitamins that affect coagulation
Vitamin K
Vitamin E

Congenital and acquired abnormalities in clotting must be identified and contingency plans made. The normal clotting cascade involves primary and secondary hemostatic mechanisms, and there is a delicate balance between factors which promote bleeding versus those that promote coagulation in the peri-operative period. When small- or medium-sized blood vessels are injured or lacerated by injury or operation, the initial transection is usually followed by intense spasm.

In addition, platelets are activated secondary to exposure to subendothelial collagen located in the injured vessel wall causing adherence and elaboration of coagulation factors, resulting in the formation of thrombin and cross linking of fibrin to form a platelet plug with cessation of bleeding after a minute or two (primary hemostasis). Subsequently, a waterfall coagulation cascade results in the conversion of fibrin to fibrin culminating in the formation of stable fibrin clot (secondary hemostasis). Counteracting the procoagulant pathway, a number of proteolytic enzymes are produced to promote inactivation of coagulation factors by a process of fibrinolysis. The balance between these systems results in a highly regulated and controlled hemostatic process. The delicate balance of this system can be adversely affected by a number of congenital coagulation defects as well as co-morbid conditions such as hepatic insufficiency, renal insufficiency, and drug treatment with clopidogrel, coumadin, aspirin, and alcohol.

The most common congenital abnormalities are hemophilia A (Factor VIII deficiency) and hemophilia B (Factor IX deficiency). Patients with these congenital defects are able to make a platelet plug by primary hemostasis but lack the ability to make a firm fibrin clot because of the defect in secondary hemostasis. Therefore, these patients must be supported through the peri-operative or peri-injury period with the infusion of commercial Factor VIII preparation or pro-thrombin complex concentrate which contains Factor IX, to maintain factor levels above 50% of normal during the peri-operative period.

Patients with hepatic insufficiency have a decrease in synthetic function of the liver with a resultant deficiency of all coagulation factors except for III and VIII. Additionally they have decreased platelet counts as a result of hypersplenism associated with portal hypertension. Moreover, the cirrhotic liver fails to adequately clear plasma activators of the fibrinolytic system, which may result in an enhanced fibrinolysis. These patients often need aggressive administration of fresh frozen plasma and platelets during the peri-operative period.

Patients with renal insufficiency differ from patients with hepatic insufficiency in that the primary defect in coagulation associated with renal disease involves primary rather than secondary hemostasis. The defect is the result of platelet dysfunction and impaired platelet vessel wall interaction. Unfortunately, platelet transfusions are of limited to no benefit because the transfused platelets are inactivated by the same toxins as the native platelets. Transfusion of cryoprecipitate and packed red blood cells has been shown to decrease the platelet defect, although the mechanism is not clear. Similar results have been seen when the hematocrit is raised by the use of recombinant erythropoietin (EPO). Desmopressin (DDAVP) has also been used to shorten bleeding times in patients with uremia.

As the population ages, the number of elderly patients undergoing surgery, as well as those who are injured, are increasing at a rapid rate. Many of these patients take clopidogrel, aspirin, coumadin, or other blood thinning agents for a variety of reasons. Elective surgery patients should discontinue anti-coagulation therapy prior to surgery for the effects of these drugs to dissipate. If the operation cannot be delayed, then administration of reversal agents such as vitamin K, prothrombin complex concentrate, platelets, recombinant activated Factor VII or fresh frozen plasma should be considered. Obviously, the risks of thrombosis versus the risks of increased bleeding must be weighed when altering the anti-coagulation status of these patients.

Coumadin, which has a half-life of approximately 40 h, acts by blocking the synthesis of vitamin K-dependent coagulation factors. Patients undergoing elective surgery can simply stop taking their coumadin several days prior to operation. On the other hand, trauma patients or patients undergoing emergency operation require active reversal with fresh frozen plasma. While vitamin K administration can reverse the effects of coumadin, the rate of correction is variable and markedly decreases the ability to recoumadinize the patient in the post-operative period. For this reason rapid correction of anti-coagulation from coumadin therapy is usually done with infusion of fresh frozen plasma using one unit of FFP to correct the PT by approximately 2 seconds.

Aspirin therapy causes anti-coagulation by inhibiting platelet function. The defect lasts for the lifespan of the platelet, which is approximately 10 days. Since the half-life of aspirin is quite short (less than 1 h), platelet transfusions are effective in reversing the defect acutely when necessary. Clopidogrel effects last for a week or more. Platelet transfusion may be used to reverse the pharmacologic effects of clopidogrel when quick reversal is required, but the half-life of the drug is 8 h and it is in a steady state in the circulation. Recombinant-activated Factor VII has been shown to reverse the platelet inhibition associated with both clopidogrel and ASA and should be considered intraoperatively if platelet transfusion is not effective.

After the pre-operative assessment, patients should be informed of the potential risks and benefits of blood transfusions and their preferences elicited. If blood loss can be anticipated, it is important to ensure that blood and blood components are available for the patients' operative procedure. If sufficient time exists, pre-admission blood collection to prevent or reduce allogeneic blood transfusion should be considered. However, it must be acknowledged that adverse outcomes such as transfusion reaction due to clerical error or bacterial contamination may still occur with the use of autologous blood transfusion. If a patient cannot tolerate pre-operative anemia or sufficient time is not available for pre-operative blood donation, then banked blood products must be used.

Intra-Operative Blood Transfusion

The decision to transfuse blood during an operation depends on the patients' underlying physiologic status as well as the amount and rate of blood loss, and physiologic derangements. The amount of blood loss is usually monitored by the anesthesiologist's observation of the amount of blood collected in suction canisters and by weighing laparotomy pads. In addition, the anesthesiologist measures hemoglobin and hematocrit levels at regular intervals during the operation. The presence of inadequate perfusion and oxygenation of vital organs is assessed by measuring blood pressure, heart rate, ECG, temperature, and blood oxygen saturation levels continuously during the procedure. When excessive blood loss is anticipated, intra-operative red blood cell recovery should be considered. While transfusion triggers have been developed for the euvolemic anemic state in the intensive care unit during the postoperative period, the data are insufficient to precisely define a trigger for blood transfusion during an operation. Certainly blood transfusion should occur if the hemoglobin level is less than 6 g/dl and usually is not necessary when the level is greater than 10 g/dl. A visual assessment of the surgical field should be conducted on a regular basis to assess for excessive microvascular bleeding (coagulopathy). If adequate intravascular volume is maintained by the infusion of crystalloids and colloids and blood loss is slow, organ perfusion can usually be maintained with hemoglobin levels as low as 6 g/dl in an otherwise healthy individual. On the other hand, if rapid blood loss results in hypotension, the decision to transfuse red cells is made by anticipating the blood loss or on evidence of hypotension rather than a laboratory result.

When massive blood transfusion is required (ten or more units of packed red blood cells), attention must be given to preventing and managing coagulopathy. Coagulopathy should be prevented by transfusing platelets and fresh frozen plasma prior to the development of microvascular bleeding, if at all possible. Platelets should be transfused if the platelet count is below 50,000 cells/ml but may also be indicated despite an apparently adequate platelet count if there is known or suspected platelet dysfunction. Additionally, when active bleeding is ongoing, fresh frozen plasma should be administered when the international normalized ratio (INR) or activated partial thromboplastin time (APTT) is elevated. Cryoprecipitate should be given when fibrinogen concentrations are less than

80 mg/dl. Recombinant-activated Factor VII may also be indicated should component therapy not result in resolution of the coagulopathy. Disturbing reports of occasional thrombotic complications leading to stroke, myocardial infarction, and intestinal ischemia after rVIIa are emerging. Therefore, this agent should be used with restraint and reserved for patients with recalcitrant coagulopathy unresponsive to component therapy.

When blood loss approaches one blood volume (approximately 70 ml/kg) a massive transfusion protocol should be initiated. This protocol does not require abnormal laboratory values as a transfusion trigger, and usually involves infusion of one unit of fresh frozen plasma and one unit of platelets for each unit of red blood cell transfused. From a practical perspective, for each unit of packed red blood cells, one unit of fresh frozen plasma should be infused along with a 6-pack of platelets for every 6 units of packed red blood cells transfused.

Special considerations must be accounted for when dealing with injured patients arriving in hemorrhagic shock as a result of blood loss prior to patient arrival. In this situation a large degree of hemorrhage has already occurred leading to impaired physiology, poor organ perfusion, and compensatory responses to preserve blood flow to the brain and heart, which are likely already at maximal capacity. As a result of marked peripheral vasoconstriction and decreased blood pressure, bleeding may have already markedly slowed or even ceased. To successfully treat these patients intravascular volume must be restored simultaneously with control of hemorrhage. Prior to definitive control of hemorrhage there is a fine line between too little fluids, resulting in hypoperfusion with organ ischemia, and too much fluid, leading to re-bleeding as a result of "popping the clot." From a practical perspective, this means transfusing packed red blood cells and crystalloid solution at a rate which is slow enough to gradually increase blood pressure towards normal, while rapidly identifying the source of hemorrhage and stopping it. The second major consideration in this group of patients is the development of coagulopathy. These patients are often cold, acidotic, and hypotensive, all of which lead to coagulopathy. Ongoing hemorrhage and massive transfusion perpetuate the acidosis and hypothermia leading to the "bloody vicious cycle" with eventual death from exsanguination. Unlike the patient undergoing elective surgery where blood loss can be easily monitored and quantified, as well as anticipated, these patients generally meet the criteria for a massive transfusion protocol at the initiation of their therapy. Laboratory values have little to do with the management of these patients. They should be transfused in a 1:1:1 ratio, receiving a unit of fresh frozen plasma for each unit of packed red blood cells and a six pack of platelets for every six units of packed red blood cells transfused.

In addition to early institution of a massive transfusion protocol, these patients require active rewarming and adherence to the principles of damage control operation. Damage control refers to limiting the operation to stopping the bleeding prior to the development of coagulopathy and terminating the procedure prior to definitive repair of all injuries. Major bleeding vessels are rapidly repaired or ligated and hollow viscus injuries are stapled closed to prevent further contamination. The abdomen is closed with a temporary closure to prevent abdominal compartment syndrome and the patient is taken to the ICU to correct abnormal physiology. The patient is returned to the operating room 24–48 h later for definitive reconstruction.

Post-Operative Blood Transfusion

Once the critical emergency or elective operation is over, and active bleeding has been controlled, the patient usually ends up in an intensive care or other monitored environment with support of their vital organs and close monitoring of their physiology. Ideally, by the end of the operation or shortly after arrival in the intensive care unit the patient has been restored to a normal euvolemic state. A variety of physiologic compensation mechanisms including regional and microcirculatory changes in blood flow and a shift of the oxyhemoglobin dissociation curve to the right to decrease hemoglobin affinity for oxygen are in place which allow adequate oxygenation of tissues at a relatively anemic but normovolemic state. Factors such as increased cardiac output and decreased blood viscosity allow oxygen delivery to remain relatively unchanged until hemoglobin concentration falls below 7 g/dl. This level is much lower than the previously recommended 10 g/dl as a transfusion trigger and is supported by the prospective randomized transfusion requirements in critical care (TRICC) trial. While there is some variability between patients it appears that the 7 g/dl trigger provides sufficient oxygen carrying capacity for all patients except those with severe coronary artery disease. Most agree that patients with known cardiovascular disease should be transfused to a higher threshold in the 8.5–10 g/dl range. Whether similar transfusion triggers should be used for patients who are elderly, have nervous system problems, COPD, or renal disease remains to be determined. Practically, transfusion guidelines should take into account the patients' individual ability to tolerate and to compensate for an acute decrease in hemoglobin concentration. As there is no "universal" hemoglobin threshold that can serve for all patients, useful transfusion triggers should consider signs of inadequate tissue oxygenation that may occur depending on the patient's underlying diseases. Physiologic signs of inadequate oxygenation such as hemodynamic instability, oxygen extraction ratio > 50%, and myocardial ischemia, detectable by new ST-segment depressions > 0.1 mV, new ST-segment elevations > 0.2 mV or new wall motion abnormalities by transesophageal echocardiography have been suggested as triggers for transfusion. Ideally, transfusion should occur prior to the development of overt signs of ischemia.

Alternatives to Blood Transfusion

Given the risks of adverse outcomes associated with blood transfusion and the finite blood supply, strategies to minimize the need for blood transfusion must be pursued. Pre-operative donation of autologous blood (ABD) and injection of recombinant human erythropoietin (EPO), along with the cessation of anticoagulant drugs are the main options. In procedures with relatively predictable blood loss such as total joint replacement surgery, ABD has been shown to decrease the percent of patients receiving an allogeneic blood transfusion. On the other hand, only 50% of the ABD blood was actually transfused in that study, calling into question its cost effectiveness. The use of pre-operative EPO has been shown to reduce the need for allogeneic blood transfusion in anemic patients, but requires one week to become effective.

The primary techniques to minimize allogeneic blood transfusion include cell salvage techniques, acceptance of minimal hemoglobin levels, aggressive hemostatic techniques, and potentially artificial oxygen carriers. Blood salvage techniques have become commonplace, appear to be safe, and reduce the volume of homologous blood transfusion, but have not decreased the number of patients receiving homologous blood transfusion. The most common adjuvant hemostatic techniques include the application of agents such as fibrin glue and thrombin in a variety of preparations. There is ongoing research in this area which holds promise for the future. The development of artificial oxygen carriers to replace red blood cell transfusion is also promising, but has been disappointing to date. There are two main groups of artificial O_2 carriers: hemoglobin-based and perfluorocarbon emulsions. The hemoglobin molecule in hemoglobin-based artificial O_2 carriers needs to be stabilized to prevent dissociation of the $alpha_2beta_2$-hemoglobin tetramer into alphabeta-dimers in order to prolong intravascular retention and to eliminate nephrotoxicity. Other modifications serve to decrease O_2 affinity in order to improve O_2 off-loading to tissues. In addition, polyethylene glycol may be surface conjugated to increase molecular size. Finally, certain products are polymerized to increase the hemoglobin concentration at physiologic colloid oncotic pressure. Perfluorocarbons are carbon-fluorine compounds characterized by a high gas-dissolving capacity for O_2 and CO_2 and chemical and biologic inertness. Perfluorocarbons are not miscible with water and therefore need to be brought into emulsion for intravenous application. The most advanced products are in clinical phase III trials, but no product has achieved market approval yet in the US, Europe, or Canada.

Post-operatively, cell salvage, EPO, and acceptance of minimal hemoglobin values represent the most common alternatives to RBC transfusion. ICU-associated anemia is largely the result of the cumulative effects of blood loss and decreased RBC production. Blood loss in critically ill patients may be overt, occult, or due to phlebotomy. Decreased RBC production is the other major factor influencing the development of anemia. Decreased RBC production is due to the combined effects of abnormal iron metabolism, inappropriately low erythropoietin production, diminished response to erythropoietin, and direct suppression of RBC production.

Clinical trials have shown that compared with non-treated subjects, rHuEPO-treated ICU patients will have increased serum erythropoietin concentrations, increased reticulocyte counts, increased hemoglobin and hematocrit values, and require fewer RBC transfusions. These clinical trials have not detected significant differences in outcomes in association with rHuEPO, however. Retransfusion of unwashed RBCs collected from drains and chest tubes has been used effectively in a variety of settings. The reported complication rate is low, but so are the total number of patients reported. When considering alternatives to red blood cell transfusion one must remember the incredibly low mortality associated with banked blood. Studies to show an equivalent safety profile with alternatives will be most challenging.

Selected Readings

Blajchman MA (2006) The clinical benefits of the leukoreduction of blood products. J Trauma 60:583–590

Hebert TC, Wells G, Blajchman MA, et al. (1999) A multicentered randomized control clinical trial of transfusion requirements in critical care. New Engl J Med 340:409–417

Practice Guidelines for Perioperative Blood Transfusion and Adjuvant Therapies (2006) An Updated Report by the American Society of Anesthesiologists Task Force on Perioperative Blood Transfusion and Adjuvant Therapies. Anesthesiology 105:198–208

Madjdpour C, et al. (2005) Perioperative blood transfusions. Value, risks, and guidelines. Anaesthesist, 54:67–80

6
Circulatory Monitoring

Eric J. Mahoney, Walter L. Biffl, and William G. Cioffi

Pearls and Pitfalls

- Normal vital signs do not equate to circulatory adequacy.
- Tachycardia indicates a loss of 15–30% of blood volume, but can be blunted in the elderly, the athlete, pregnant women, and patients medicated with beta-blockers. Automated blood pressure devices lack accuracy when the systolic blood pressure is below 110 mmHg; use of a manual device in these settings is recommended.
- Monitor the mean arterial pressure (MAP), NOT the systolic blood pressure.
- Measure central venous pressure (CVP) and pulmonary capillary wedge pressure (PCWP) at end expiration.
- Beware that base deficits and lactic acidosis do not always occur secondary to hypoxia.
- Use oxygen delivery (DO2) as a guide, not as an endpoint.

Introduction

The fundamental goal of circulatory monitoring is to assess the adequacy of tissue perfusion. At first glance, this would appear to be relatively straightforward – heart rate and blood pressure are easy to assess and to interpret. However, neither accurately reflects perfusion, and the assessment of circulatory

K.I. Bland et al. (eds.), *General Principles of Surgery*,
DOI 10.1007/978-1-84996-381-7_6,
© Springer-Verlag London Limited 2011

adequacy becomes much more difficult with increasing severity or complexity of illness. With several methods available to evaluate a patient's circulatory status, the clinician must learn to utilize and to interpret various monitoring modalities. In this chapter, we will discuss each of these methods (Table 6.1).

TABLE 6.1. Means of circulatory monitoring.

	Advantages	Disadvantages
Physical examination	Simple	Non-specific insensitive
Pulse	Accessible reliable	Age variation
		Influenced by:
		Medications
		Physiological status
		Insensitive to occult hypoperfusion
Noninvasive blood pressure monitoring (sphygmomanometry)	Accessible	Unreliable
	Good indicator of vital organ perfusion	Insensitive to occult
		hypoperfusion
		Influenced by:
		Poor cuff fit
		Limitations to auscultation
		Atherosclerosis
Invasive blood pressure monitoring (arterial lines)	Accurate	Invasive
	Continuous blood pressure	Infectious risk

(continued)

TABLE 6.I. (continued)

	Advantages	Disadvantages
	Monitoring	Thrombosis/ischemic risk
	Access for blood tests	System malfunction
		Transducer height
		Dampening
		Mismatching
		Catheter whip
Pulmonary artery catheters	Assess volume status	Invasive
	Assess left heart function	Infectious risk
	Assess oxygen delivery (DO_2) and	Thrombosis/embolism risk
	oxygen uptake (VO_2)	
		Cardiac conduction risks:
		Arrhythmias
		Complete heart block
		Ventricular perforation
		Pulmonary artery rupture
		Misinterpretation
Central venous pressure monitoring	Assess volume status	Invasive
	Assess right heart function	Infectious risk
		System malfunction

(continued)

TABLE 6.I. (continued)

	Advantages	Disadvantages
		Pneumothorax
		Hemothorax
		Chylothorax
		Brachial plexus injury
		Mediastinitis
		Affect by premorbid cardiac and pulmonary conditions
Serum lactic acid	Assess global perfusion	Non-specific
Serum base deficit	Assess global perfusion	Non-specific

Physical Examination

Circulatory monitoring begins with the physical examination. Frequently, important signs will be noticed within the first 10 seconds of the examination. Although many of the signs discovered may be non-specific, taken as a whole they provide valuable information regarding the status of the patient. During severe circulatory compromise, a patient may be very anxious, confused, or obtunded. Jugular venous distension is a common sign of cardiogenic shock or volume overload. Increased sympathetic tone leads to tachycardia as well as peripheral vasoconstriction with associated cool, clammy skin. Dry mucous membranes, sunken eyes, and decreased skin turgor are signs of chronic hypovolemia. Additionally, decreased urine output in a patient is a compensatory mechanism whereby water excretion is minimized in an attempt to maintain blood volume. These physical characteristics must be elucidated by the examiner and properly evaluated with the objective information presented in order to treat the patient properly.

Pulse

The pulse should be assessed for rate, rhythm, and strength. The normal heart rate varies with age (Table 6.2). Tachycardia is a fairly reliable marker of circulatory compromise. It may be a response to hypovolemia or cardiac ischemia; or it may also be a cause of circulatory compromise when a brief diastolic interval precludes adequate cardiac filling. In most cases, tachycardia and cutaneous vasoconstriction are early and predictable physiologic responses to hypovolemia. The appearance of tachycardia indicates a loss of 15–30% of circulating blood volume. With increasing blood loss, there is a progressive increase in heart rate and respiratory rate (Table 6.3). An abnormal rhythm may also signify cardiac ischemia or be

TABLE 6.2. Normal pulse rate variations with age.

Age (years)	Infant	2–6	7–13	Adult (>13)
Normal pulse range (bpm)	140–160	120–140	100–120	60–100

TABLE 6.3. Estimated fluid and blood losses based on patient's presentation (Adapted from American College of Surgeons' Committee on Trauma, 2004. With permission).

	CLASS 1	CLASS 2	CLASS 3	CLASS 4
Blood loss (ml)	Up to 750	750–1,500	1,500–2,000	>2,000
Blood loss (% blood volume)	Up to 15%	15–30%	30–40%	>40%
Pulse rate (bpm)	<100	>100	>120	>140
Blood pressure (mmHg)	Normal	Normal	Decreased	Decreased
Respiratory rate	14–20	20–30	30–40	>40
Urine output (ml/h)	>30	20–30	5–15	Negligible
CNS/Mental status	Slightly anxious	Mildly anxious	Anxious, confused	Confused, lethargic
Fluid replacement (3:1 rule)	Crystalloid	Crystalloid	Crystalloid and blood	Crystalloid and blood

TABLE 6.4. Approximate minimal systolic blood pressures based on palpable pulse locations.

Pulse location	Radial	Brachial	Femoral	Carotid
Approximate SBP (mmHg)	90	80	70	60

associated with compromised cardiac output, such as is the case with rapid atrial fibrillation or flutter. Whereas a strong distal pulse is reassuring, a thready pulse signifies circulatory compromise. The minimal systolic blood pressure may be estimated by the anatomic location of a palpable pulse (Table 6.4). Finally, asymmetry of pulses is typical of pathologic processes such as atherosclerotic stenosis, arterial dissection, or other pathology.

One should be mindful of special circumstances during which the expected physiological responses to inadequate circulation may not be apparent. For example the elderly may be unable to mount the expected increase in heart rate or inotropy in order to respond to shock due to a decrease in sympathetic tone and reserve. Additionally, the use of beta-adrenergic antagonist medication or a cardiac pacemaker in this cohort of patients may prevent the tachycardic response to hemorrhage. Also, in young healthy athletic adults and in pregnant women, physiological adaptations result in a markedly expanded blood volume. Thus, relatively large amounts of blood loss may result in only modest elevations in heart rate. This relative hypervolemia provides an additional compensatory mechanism for the individual and limits the elevation in heart rate until a profound volume of blood is lost.

Blood Pressure

Non-invasive (Sphygmomanometry)

The blood pressure cuff is applied to a limb, usually the upper arm, and is inflated to a pressure that eliminates flow in the underlying artery as determined by auscultation or palpation of loss of a pulse. When the cuff is deflated and cuff pressure falls below systolic pressure, blood begins to flow through the artery again, but in turbulent fashion. This first audible sound is designated the systolic blood pressure. As the cuff is deflated, the artery will no longer be compressed, and flow will become laminar again and no longer be audible. The pressure at which this occurs is designated the diastolic pressure.

The clinician must be wary of relying too heavily on sphygmomanometry for patient care. The arterial blood pressure "is one of the most common and most unreliable measurements in modern medicine." Cuff pressures can be misleading because this mode relies on the assumption that pressures in the cuff are the same as those in the encompassed artery. While this assumption is usually correct, errors often occur as the result of inappropriately sized cuffs. Although seldom checked, the length of the bladder of the cuff should be at least 80% of the circumference of the upper arm, and the width at least 40% of the circumference of the upper arm in order for the measurement to be accurate. If the bladder is too small, blood pressure measurements will be erroneously high; if too big, erroneously low. Patients with atherosclerotic disease may have falsely elevated readings due to non-compressible, calcified arteries. In the morbidly obese, due to a conical rather than cylindrical shape of the arm or a poor fit of the blood pressure cuff pressure, the readings may be falsely elevated. Furthermore, due to limitation on human hearing, listening for sounds generated from the artery (Korotkoff sounds) as the cuff deflates can be very inaccurate, especially during hypotension. On the other hand, automated blood pressure cuffs are not consistently accurate when systolic blood pressures are below 110 mmHg (American College of Surgeons' Committee on Trauma, 2004). For these reasons, direct intravascular monitoring may be preferred in critically ill patients.

Invasive (Arterial Lines)

Arterial lines are an invasive means of monitoring blood pressure that require the cannulation of an artery, but provide real-time assessment of the blood pressure. Indications for arterial line insertion include the need for continuous arterial pressure monitoring, arterial blood gas monitoring, and access for frequent blood tests. Although an improvement over sphygmomanometry, arterial lines too, can be inaccurate. After the artery is cannulated and the pressure transducer is calibrated, the transducer must be zeroed at the level of the right atrium or else reading will be erroneous: falsely elevated if the transducer is too low, falsely depressed if the transducer is too high.

The measured systolic pressure may be inaccurate due to mismatching between the catheter and the artery, catheter whip, or reflected pressure waves. Mismatching refers to the compliance of the catheter relative to the arterial wall. If the catheter tubing is too stiff compared to the artery, the systolic pressure will be higher and the diastolic lower than the actual pressure in the artery. Conversely, if the tubing is more compliant than the vessel, dampening of the pressure will occur, and the measured systolic pressure will be lower and the diastolic pressure higher. Catheter whip is due to movement of the catheter within the lumen of the vessel. This usually occurs when the catheter is placed in a relatively large vessel, such as the femoral artery, and can cause the measurements of systolic pressure to vary by approximately 20 mmHg. The systolic pressure is normally amplified in the periphery due to pressure waves being reflected back centrally from vascular bifurcations and stenotic vessels. As pathophysiologic atherosclerotic changes occur in the vessels, this amplification will be more pronounced and systolic pressures will be falsely elevated. Also, severe peripheral vasoconstriction may lower pressure in the distal arteries compared to the proximal arteries. Given these potential inaccuracies, it is wise to follow – and titrate therapy – to the mean arterial pressure, as it is relatively consistent throughout the vasculature and should be considered accurate.

Cannulation of an artery is not a completely benign procedure and can lead to serious complications. These include catheter-related bloodstream infections, pseudoaneurysms, and thromboembolism. The latter may lead to distal ischemia or necrosis. Therefore arterial catheters should be inserted in arteries with considerable collateral circulation, such as the radial artery, rather than brachial artery. Because ischemia of the hand is functionally devastating, one should always assess collateral circulation of the radial artery before cannulation by performing an Allen's test. Continuous intraarterial fluid infusion may also be employed to prevent catheter thrombosis.

Central Venous Pressure Monitoring

Central venous pressure (CVP) monitoring involves the measurement of pressure in a central vein (e.g. vena cava, subclavian vein, jugular vein). Although pressure does not always equate to volume, CVP is used to assess preload as well as right heart function. The transducer must be placed at the zero reference point, known as the phlebostatic axis, for central venous pressures to be accurate. This phlebostatic axis is the artificial point on the thorax where the fourth intercostal space meets the midaxillary line, and corresponds to the position of the right and left atria in the supine position.

Since the intrathoracic pressure varies with the respiratory cycle, the most accurate CVP measurement is made at end-expiration when the vascular transmural pressures approach zero. The practitioner must account for positive end-expiratory pressure (PEEP) in patients who are being mechanically ventilated because this may elevate the measured CVP. Alternatively, if the patient can tolerate it, the CVP may be measured with the PEEP temporarily discontinued.

Although the "normal" CVP is quoted as between 4–8 mmHg, the optimal CVP for circulatory adequacy depends on the function of the heart. In general, a sick patient with a low CVP (0–4 mmHg) usually benefits from volume resuscitation, and a patient with a "normal" CVP (4–8 mmHg) may or may not benefit from additional fluid. When the CVP is > 8 mmHg, the clinician may need to use additional means to assess the circulatory adequacy and then make a therapeutic decision. Of particular significance is the change in CVP over time, e.g. after fluid resuscitation, and what affect this has on cardiac function,

TABLE 6.5. Factors leading to elevated CVP.

Acute left sided myocardial infarction
Diseases with ejection fraction < 50%
Mitral or tricuspid value regurgitation
Pulmonary embolism
Tension pneumothorax
Pericardial tamponade

vital signs, tissue perfusion, and overall clinical status. Only a change of CVP of greater than 4 mmHg is considered clinically significant.

In a patient with normal cardiac function, CVP approximates the pulmonary capillary wedge pressure, which in turn approximates the left atrial end-diastolic pressure. However, there are multiple acute and chronic cardiac and pulmonary diseases that interfere with this relationship. These are listed in Table 6.5. In these cases, simultaneous assessment of right and left heart function with a pulmonary artery catheter may be helpful (see below).

When deciding to monitor CVP one must consider the risks of inserting a CVP catheter into the internal jugular or subclavian vein. These include pneumothorax, hemothorax, chylothorax, brachial plexus injury, and mediastinitis. Several studies have shown that ultrasound guided placement of intravenous catheters is the safest method of placement.

Pulmonary Artery Catheters (Pac)

Pulmonary artery catheters are useful in assessing the filling pressures of the left and right sides of the heart and in providing objective data on cardiac performance. These long catheters (110 cm in length) are passed through a central venous introducer or cordis and then "floated" into the right heart and pulmonary artery with the assistance of an inflatable balloon located just proximal to the tip of the catheter. The balloon

TABLE 6.6. Clinical data available from pulmonary artery catheters (Adapted from Marino, 1998).

Central venous pressure	Stroke volume index
Pulmonary artery pressure	Left ventricular stroke work index
Pulmonary capillary wedge pressure	Right ventricular stroke work index
Cardiac output	Right ventricular ejection fraction
Cardiac index	Systemic vascular resistance
Oxygen delivery	Pulmonary vascular resistance
Oxygen uptake	Mixed venous oxygen saturation
Oxygen extraction ratio	

can then be "wedged" in a smaller pulmonary artery. From the pulmonary artery catheter, a large amount of information can be obtained (Table 6.6). Since the measuring port of the catheter lies just distal to the balloon, and taking into account the valveless pulmonary venous system, the pulmonary capillary wedge pressure approximates the left atrial pressure (except in cases of pulmonary hypertension) which will equal left-ventricular end diastolic pressure in patients with competent mitral valves.

One value that can be extrapolated from the PAC is the Oxygen Delivery (DO_2). This is defined as the product of the oxygen content and the cardiac output (CO):

$$DO_2 = CO \times 13:4 \times Hemoglobin \times SaO_2$$

Oxygen delivery is typically reported as an indexed value (normal range 520–570 ml $O_2/min/m^2$); thus the cardiac index is used in the calculation. Also, one can calculate Oxygen Consumption (VO_2), which is defined as the difference in oxygen content between the arterial and mixed venous blood:

$$VO_2 = CO \times 13:4 \times Hemoglobin (g/dl) \times (SaO_2 \times SvO_2)$$

The normal range for indexed VO_2 is 110–160 ml O_2/min/m^2. The ratio of the Oxygen Consumption to Oxygen Delivery is called the Oxygen Extraction Ratio (O_2ER):

$$O_2ER = (VO_2 / DO_2) \times 100$$

The normal range for O_2ER is 20–30%. However, this is highly variable. When metabolic demands are increased or when oxygen delivery falls, the VO_2 increases and the O_2ER can reach 50–60% in order to maintain aerobic metabolism.

Previously, Shoemaker and colleagues identified values for cardiac index (4.5 l/min/m^2), DO_2 (600 ml O_2/min/m^2) and VO_2 (170 ml O_2/min/m^2) above which survival could be predicted in critically ill patients. However, subsequent randomized controlled trials by other researchers using these as endpoints of resuscitation were mixed as to any survivor benefit. In support of the aforementioned research, Shoemaker and Kern published a meta-analysis of randomized controlled trials that had evaluated resuscitation to normal or supranormal values. They concluded that successful resuscitation to supranormal physiologic values resulted in a significant reduction in organ failure and mortality but only among the most severely injured (i.e. those with > 20% predicted mortality) and when initiated prior to the onset of organ failure. These results are supported by Boyd whose metaanalysis of six randomized studies concluded that there was an improvement in outcome, but again only when PAC-directed therapy was initiated prior to organ failure or sepsis. Balogh and colleagues cautioned that supranormal resuscitation was associated with a higher 24 h lactated Ringer's infusion requirement, with an increased incidence of abdominal compartment syndrome, multiple organ failure and mortality. Moreover, supranormal DO_2 values do not ensure adequate oxygen utilization. Moore et al. reported on a cohort of severely injured patients in whom a supranormal VO_2 was unattainable despite a supranormal DO_2. This group had a higher incidence of multiple organ failure that was theorized to be due to defective aerobic metabolism.

The Mixed Venous Oxygen Saturation (SvO_2) is the concentration of oxygen within the pulmonary artery and represents a mixture of blood returning from all parts of the body. As such, it is used as an indicator of global perfusion. The normal SvO_2 is approximately 75%. As with any physiologic variable of tissue oxygenation, it is nonspecific and is a function of oxygenation by the lungs, oxygen delivery by the cardiovascular system, and oxygen uptake by the tissues. A drop in SvO_2 could be due to deterioration in cardiac or pulmonary function, or an increase in O_2 consumption. On the other hand, the SvO_2 may be elevated in situations such as septic shock due to impaired tissue extraction and utilization of oxygen. Not even a normal SvO_2 ensures adequate oxygenation, and some advocate for concomitant lactic acid levels.

Consequently, the SvO_2 value is most helpful when it is (a) initially corroborated with another measure of perfusion, such as lactic acid; and (b) followed continuously over time. Technology exists now that provides real-time SvO_2 measurements utilizing specialized PACs that have a continuous SvO_2 monitor at the tip of the catheter. Any sudden or significant change in SvO_2 provides an early warning of a worsening condition and should prompt an aggressive search for its cause.

Similar to any invasive catheter, PACs are associated with risks such as bacterial contamination, thrombosis, and embolism. However, there are additional complications that are unique to PACs. During the manipulation of the catheter, ventricular dysrhythmias can be triggered, as well as valvular injury induced. In a patient with a pre-existing left bundle branch block, the catheter can lead to complete heart block by interfering with the right bundle branch conduction. Also, case reports of intracardiac catheter knotting have been reported.

The severe bleeding risks associated with PACs deserve special mention. The first is right ventricular perforation, which occurs due to overly aggressive insertion and can lead to pericardial tamponade and possibly death. The other is rupture of the pulmonary artery itself. This occurs when the balloon is placed (or migrates) too distally into the pulmonary artery or when the balloon is over inflated. The rupture presents suddenly as hemoptysis either during or immediately after inflation of the catheter balloon, and often mandates emergent thoracotomy with lung resection. Risk factors include pulmonary artery hypertension, advanced age, lung cancer, and coagulopathies (Bishop et al., 1993).

In addition to the risks of technical complications, several recent trials have questioned the clinical benefit of PACs. On the other hand, it has been suggested that the fault lies not with the PAC but with the interpretation of the data that it provides. The PAC is a tool with value primarily in patients whose clinical response to CVP-directed therapy is unexpected or in whom specific objective measures of cardiac performance are desired in order to direct inotropic or vasopressor therapy.

Serum Lactate

With hypoperfusion, aerobic metabolism cannot occur and anaerobic metabolism ensues. Pyruvate is therefore converted into lactic acid rather than being shunted into the tricarboxylic acid cycle. This lactic acid is released into the bloodstream and can be measured as an indicator of global perfusion. Multiple studies have demonstrated that elevated blood lactate is a reliable marker of hypoperfusion. Furthermore, failure to clear the lactate level to normal levels with 24 h was associated with a mortality of >75%.

One disadvantage of relying on blood serum lactate is that factors other than hypoperfusion may cause lactic acidosis. Lactic acidosis is classified as either Type A, Type B, or D-lactic acidosis. Type A includes syndromes associated with inadequate oxygen delivery, whereas type B lactic acidosis typically represents conditions during which lactic acidosis exists in the absence of hypoperfusion. A complete list is shown in Table 6.7.

TABLE 6.7. Lactic acidosis.

Type A
Circulatory insufficiency (shock, heart failure)
Severe anemia
Cholera
Mitochondrial enzyme defects
Carbon monoxide poisoning
Cyanide poisoning
Type B
Hypoglycemia (glycogen storage diseases)
Seizures
Diabetes mellitus
Ethanol
Severe hepatic insufficiency
Malignancy
Salicylates
Severe exercise
D-lactic acidosis
Short gut syndrome
Jejuno-ileal bypass operation

Base Deficit

The Base deficit is a measure of the number of millimoles of base required to correct the pH of a liter of whole blood to 7.40. The normal range of base deficit is þ 3 to –3 mmol/l. One may calculate the base deficit from the arterial blood gas as follows:

If $PaCO_2 < 40$

Ideal $PaCO_2$ (i.e. 40) – measured $PaCO_2 = \Delta PaCO_2$
Then $\Delta PaCO_2 \times 0{:}008 =$ calculated ΔpH

Then (7:40 + calculated ΔpH) – measured pH = actual ΔpH
Then actual ΔpH $\times$ 2/3 $\times$ 100 = Base deficit

If $PaCO_2 > 40$

Measured $PaCO_2$ – Ideal $PaCO_2$ (i.e. 40) = $\Delta PaCO_2$
Then $\Delta PaCO_2 \times 0.008$ = calculated ΔpH
Then (7:40 – calculated ΔpH) – measured pH = actual ΔpH
Then actual Δ pH $\times$ 2/3 $\times$ 100 = Base deficit

Early on during hypovolemia, base deficit can be used as an indirect measurement of lactic acidosis. In seminal work done by Davis and colleagues (Davis et al., 1991), base deficit was shown to correlate with volume requirement as well as being a sensitive indicator of severity of shock and efficacy of resuscitation. However, the base deficit lacks specificity, and any condition that leads to acidemia (e.g. renal tubular acidosis, diabetic ketoacidosis) will lead to elevations in the base deficit.

Summary

Assessment of circulatory adequacy is an integral component of surgical care. Physical examination and assessment of vital signs may detect more profound circulatory deficits. However, there is a role for more invasive monitoring in critically ill patients. In complex patients who may be susceptible to occult hypoperfusion, monitoring of global indicators of perfusion can help guide resuscitation.

Selected Readings

Abramson D, Scalea TM, Hitchcock R, et al. (1993) Lactate clearance and survival following injury. J Trauma 35:584–588

American College of Surgeons' Committee on Trauma (2004) Advanced Trauma Life Support for Doctors (ATLS) Student manual, 7th edn. American College of Surgeons, Chicago, IL

Balogh Z, McKinley MA, Cocanour CS, et al. (2003) Supranormal trauma resuscitation causes more cases of abdominal compartment syndrome. Arch Surg 138:637–642

Bishop MH, Shoemaker WC, Appel PL, et al. (1993) Relationship between supranormal circulatory values, time delays, and outcomes in severely traumatized patients. Crit Care Med 21:56–63

Boyd O (2000) The high risk surgical patient: where are we now? Clin Intensive Care Special Issue:3–10

Burchard KW, Gann DS, Wiles CE (2000) The circulation, ch. 2. In: Burchard KW, Gann DS, Wiles CE (eds) The clinical handbook for surgical critical care. Parthenon, New York

Davis JW, Davis IC, Bennink LD, et al. (2003) Are automated blood pressure measurements accurate in trauma patients? J Trauma 55:860–863

Davis JW, Shackford SR, Holbrook TL (1991) Base deficit as a sensitive indicator of compensated shock and tissue oxygen utilization. Surg Gynecol Obstet 173:473

Davis JW, Shackford SR, Mackersie RC, et al. (1988) Base deficit as a guide to volume resuscitation. J. Trauma 28:146

DuBose, Thomas Jr D (1998) Acidosis and alkalosis, ch. 50. In: Fauci AS, Braunwald E, Isselbacher KJ, et al. (eds) Harrison's principles of internal medicine, 14th edn. McGraw Hill, New York, pp 279–280

Elliott DC (1998) An evaluation of the endpoints of resuscitation. J Am Coll Surg 187:536–547

Friedman G, et al. (1995) Combined measurements of blood lactate concentrations and gastric intramucosal pH in patients with severe sepsis. Crit Care Med 23:1184–1193

Marino PL (1998) Hemodynamic monitoring, sec. 3. In: Marino PL (ed) The ICU book, 2nd edn. Williams & Wilkins, Baltimore, MD

Holcroft JW, Anderson JT (2005) Cardiopulmonary monitoring, sec. 6, ch. 4. In: American College of Surgeons (eds) ACS surgery principles and practice. WebMD Publishing, New York

Iberti TJ, et al. (1990) A multicenter study of physicians' knowledge of the pulmonary artery catheter. JAMA 264:2928–2932

Keenan, SP (2002) Use of ultrasound to place central lines. J Crit Care 17:126–137

Kern JW, Shoemaker WC (2002) Meta-analysis of hemodynamic optimization in high-risk patients. Crit Care Med 30:1686–1692

Moore FA, Haenel JB, Moore EE, et al. (1992) Incommensurate oxygen consumption in response to maximal oxygen availability predicts post-injury multiple organ failure. J Trauma 33:58–66

Shah MR et al. (2005) Impact of the pulmonary artery catheter in critically ill patients: meta-analysis of randomized clinical trials. JAMA 294:1664–1670

7

Acute Pain Management

Edmund A.M. Neugebauer

Pearls and Pitfalls

- Sufficient pain management is a prerequisite for enhanced patient recovery and for a reduction in postoperative morbidity and mortality.
- Pain assessment and documentation ("fifth vital sign") are fundamental prerequisites for adequate pain management.
- Opioids remain the fundamental group of analgesic drugs for the treatment of moderate to severe pain.
- Co-analgesics support the action of analgesics but are not sufficient alone for postoperative pain relief.
- Peripheral nerve blocks have the advantage of not compromising patient alertness.
- Local analgesics are very effective in epidural analgesia.
- Epidural local anesthetics lead to a decreased incidence of pulmonary infection and complications overall compared with opioids.
- Treatment of acute pain should be procedure-specific and treatment should be adapted to the measured pain intensity reported by the patient.
- Pain management is an interdisciplinary task requiring close liaison with all personnel involved in the care of the patient.
- Use of evidence-based clinical practice guidelines are recommended and should be adapted locally.

K.I. Bland et al. (eds.), *General Principles of Surgery*, 109
DOI 10.1007/978-1-84996-381-7_7,
© Springer-Verlag London Limited 2011

"Acute pain management is a basic human right."

(Professor M. I. Cousins, President, Australian and New Zealand College of Anaesthetists)

Although major efforts have been conducted to improve acute pain management in recent years, we are still far away in meeting this basic human right. In the USA and Europe, the results of studies dedicated specifically to both medical and postoperative patients in academic hospitals have shown unequivocally that pain remains undertreated. Pain should not be an accompanying phenomenon of medical treatments; in principle, the possibilities for adequate pain management are available to all. Sufficient pain therapy is an important prerequisite for enhanced patient recovery and will reduce the postoperative risk of morbidity and mortality. Moreover, a significant reduction in long-term morbidity can be achieved since moderate to severe pain has been demonstrated as an independent predictor for chronic postoperative pain. Adequate pain therapy is cost-effective; it is associated with a decrease in both intensive care and overall hospital stay. Studies have shown that up to 70% of patients present to hospital because of acute pain. Furthermore, they associate the success of medical treatment with the relief of pain and it is of significant value from the patients' perspective.

Definition

Pain as defined by the International Association for the Study of Pain is "an unpleasant sensory and emotional experience associated with actual or potential tissue damage, or described in terms of such damage." Pain is subjective and is an individual, multifactorial experience influenced by culture, previous pain events, mood, beliefs, and an ability to cope. *Acute pain* is defined as "pain of recent onset and probable limited duration." It usually has an identifiable temporal and causal relationship to injury (trauma, operation) or disease (colic, peritonitis, etc.). *Chronic pain* persists commonly beyond the time of healing of an injury (>3–6 months) and frequently has no clear identifiable cause. Acute and chronic pain may represent a continuum.

Pathophysiological and Pharmacological Basics

Pain development and transduction involves multiple interacting peripheral and central mechanisms. The understanding of principles is important for the choice of medical treatments and will therefore be summarized briefly. The basis of each central nervous system function is the excitation–response relationship.

Peripheral level: Acute pain starts by tissue injury caused by mechanical, thermal, or chemical excitation. The detection of noxious stimuli requires activation of peripheral sensory organs (nociceptors) and transduction of the energy into electrical signals for conduction to the central nervous system. Nociceptive afferents are distributed widely throughout the body (skin, muscle, joints, viscera, meninges).

Spinal cord level: Once transducted into electrical stimuli, conduction of neuronal action potentials into afferent input and dorsal horn output follows. This signal conduction is called transmission in the spinal cord. The processing of pain on its way from excitation to perception is subject to several transformations. Tissue damage such as that associated with infection, inflammation, or ischemia, produces an array of chemical mediators (algetic substances such as prostaglandins, and histamines) that can sensitize nociceptors to increase pain perception. This increase in sensitivity is termed peripheral sensitization, which can also lead to central sensitization. In addition to the excitatory processes, inhibitory modulation occurs within the dorsal horn.

Central projecting level: A peripheral pain signal, which reaches the central nervous system after transduction, transmission, and transformation needs to be translated into pain perception. The areas of the brain involved are the limbic system, cortex (e.g. cingulate cortex, insula, prefrontal cortex), and thalamus. The perception and experience of pain is multifactorial and is further influenced by psychological and environmental factors of each individual. Figure 7.1 gives a schematic representation of the nociceptor pathway.

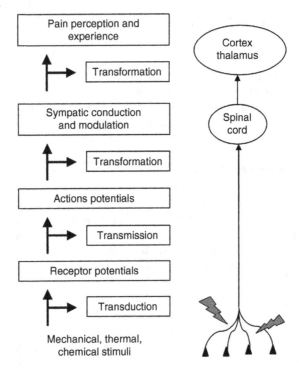

FIGURE 7.1. Overview of the nociceptor pathway.

TABLE 7.1. Categories of analgesic drugs.

Non-opioids

Opioids

Local anesthetics

Co-analgesics

Adjuvant drugs

For adequate pain management, it is necessary to be familiar with the main mechanisms of pain relief by the different analgesic drugs (Table 7.1 and Fig. 7.2). Analgesic drugs can be subdivided into five major categories.

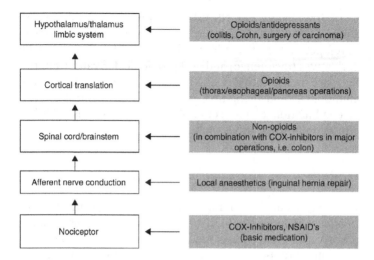

FIGURE 7.2. Nociceptive pathway and therapeutic options of pain relief.

Non-opioid Analgesics

The basic action of most non-opioids (nonsteroidal anti-inflammatory drugs – NSAIDs) is the inhibition of the cyclooxygenase (COX) enzymes. Two subtypes of COX enzymes have been identified–the constitutive COX-1 and the "inducible" COX-2, and now a COX-3 is being investigated. Many of the effects of NSAIDs can be explained by inhibition of prostaglandin synthesis in peripheral tissues, nerves, and the central nervous system. Prostaglandins have many physiological functions including gastric mucosal protection, renal tubular function, intrarenal vasodilatation, bronchodilatation, and production of endothelial prostacyclin. Such physiological roles are mainly regulated by COX-1 and are a basis for many of the adverse effects associated with NSAID use. Tissue damage results in COX-2 production, leading to synthesis of prostaglandins that result in pain and inflammation. NSAIDs are nonselective COX inhibitors that inhibit both COX-1 and COX-2 with a wide spectrum of analgesic, antiinflammatory, antipyretic effects. Aspirin acetylates inhibit

COX irreversibly but NSAIDs are reversible inhibitors of enzymes. The COX-2 inhibitors (e.g., parecoxib) have been developed to selectively inhibit the inducible form. Arylacid derivatives (diclofenac) and aryl propionic derivates (ibuprofen) are nonselective COX-inhibitors. Paracetamol (acetaminophen) and metamizol have additional central effects. A combination of paracetamol and NSAIDs has additive effects on postoperative analgesia.

Opioids

Opioids remain the central group of analgesic drugs for the treatment of moderate to severe acute pain and transmit their action via different types of receptors. Opioids can be differentiated into pure μ-agonists (morphine, oxycodone, fentanyl, tramadole), mixed agonists–antagonists (antagonistic at μ-receptors and agonistic at k- and s-receptors, e.g., pentazocin, tilidine), partial agonists with high affinity and small intrinsic activity at μ-receptors (buprenorphine), and pure antagonists (at μ-, κ-, and δ-receptors) such as naloxone.

The opioid receptors are located mostly at structures that are involved in transmission, transformation, and translation of afferent signals. A high density is found in the limbic system, the thalamus, the pons region, and the substancia gelatinosa in the dorsal horn. Clinically meaningful side effects are dose-related; once a threshold dose is reached, every 3–4 mg increase of morphine-equivalent dose per day is associated with one additional adverse event. The most significant adverse effects are sedation, pruritus, nausea, and vomiting. The risk can be reduced significantly by parallel application of NSAIDs and/or adjuvant drugs. In the management of acute pain one opioid is not superior to others but some opioids appear more effective in some patients than others.

Local Anesthetics

Local anesthetics exert their effects as analgesics by impeding neuronal excitation and/or conduction. Short-duration local

anesthetics (lignocaine, plasma half-life 90 m) have to be differentiated from long-duration local anesthetics (bupivacaine, ropivacaine). The local anesthetic effect depends very much on the site of administration, the dose administered, and the presence or absence of vasoconstrictors. Local application of 20 ml 0.25% bupivacaine in the area of trocar incision sites in laparoscopic cholecystectomy or colectomy reduces postoperative pain intensity significantly.

Local anesthetics are very effective in epidural analgesia. The quality of pain relief from low-dose epidural infusion (bupivacaine 0.1%, ropivacaine 0.2%) is improved consistently from the addition of adjuvants such as opioids. The concept of fast-track recovery benefits most from the application of an epidural.

Co-Analgesics and Adjuvant Drugs

Co-analgesics support the action of analgesics but are not sufficient alone for postoperative pain management. However, they are extremely helpful in combination with opioids and NSAIDs, and can reduce postoperative analgesic requirements (Table 7.2). Adjuvant drugs are mainly used to decrease side effects of analgesic drugs such as emesis, vomiting, and constipation.

Assessment and Documentation of Acute Pain

Pain assessment and documentation are fundamental prerequisites for adequate pain management. Regular assessment leads to improved pain management. Under routine clinical conditions measurement of pain intensity is sufficient and should be performed by visual analogue or numerical rating scales. Self-reporting of pain should be used whenever appropriate as pain is by definition, a subjective experience. In the pre- and postoperative setting scoring should include static

TABLE 7.2. Co-analgesics and their main functions.

Antidepressant	Increase function of inhibitory transmitter (e.g., serotonin, noradrenalin) (i.e., aminotryptiline)
Anticonvulsive	Supportive in neuropathic pain syndromes (e.g., carbamacepine, gabapentine)
Muscle relaxant	Supportive in muscle pain and spasms (e.g., benzodiazepine)
Corticosteroid	Anti-inflammatory (e.g., dexamethasone)
Bisphosphonate	Supporative in bony pain syndromes after metastasis of tumors (e.g., clodronate, pamidronate)

(rest) and dynamic (pain on sitting, coughing) measurements at least two times a day and following treatment of pain to determine efficacy. The score should be documented in the patient's charts as the "fifth vital sign." Uncontrolled or unexpected pain requires reassessment of the diagnosis and consideration of alternative causes for pain.

General Pain Management Procedures

The surgeon has a special responsibility in the treatment of pain. Aside from pharmacological interventions, consideration should be given to the possibility of intervention before, during, and after surgery to optimize pain management.

Preoperatively, the surgeon has to provide procedural information to the patient that summarizes what will happen during treatment and it is necessary to obtain sensory experiences from the patient (patient expectations). Combined sensory and procedural information is effective in reducing negative effect and reports of procedure-related pain and anxiety. The placebo-effect plays an important role and should be used. Patient information and training regarding coping and relaxation strategies have been shown to reduce pain and distress. The patients should be convinced that their pain is of utmost importance to the treating team and that they can also contribute to the success of pain management (patient as partner/co-therapist).

Intraoperatively, all treatments to the patient should be performed under the philosophy of avoiding pain wherever possible (minimal invasive techniques, positioning, etc). Drains should be avoided and wound closure should be performed preferably with absorbable sutures.

Postoperatively, a whole array of preventive measures should be considered with respect to reducing pain and associated complications: early rehabilitation (fast-track), wound management, physiotherapy, cold/heat massage techniques, and removal of lines and drains as soon as possible.

Medical Pain Management Procedures

Peripheral Nerve Blockade

The main advantage of using peripheral nerve blockade techniques as compared to systemic drug therapy is that the use of local anesthetics does not compromise patient alertness and allows pain-free mobilization.

Peripheral nerve blocks may be used for diagnostic and therapeutic purposes. Important technical issues include the technique of nerve location, the type of catheter equipment, the amount of drug, and the duration of drug efficacy. Following diagnostic location of the nerve, a continuous blockade can be undertaken. Local anesthetics such as lidocaine, mepivocaine, or prilocaine have a 2 h duration of efficacy whereas bupivacaine and ropivacaine can produce pain relief for up to 12 h. Adjuvant techniques may prolong the duration of action. For example, wound infiltration with a long-acting local anesthetic agent provides effective analgesia following inguinal hernia repair but not for open cholecystectomy or hysterectomy. Continuous femoral nerve blockade provides postoperative analgesia and functional recovery superior to intravenous morphine with fewer side effects and is comparable to epidural analgesia following knee-joint replacement surgery.

Both single injection and continuous application carry the risk of neurological injury, intravascular injection, dislodgment, hematoma, and infection. The incidence of neurological injury following peripheral nerve blocks is 0.02–0.4%.

Epidural Analgesia

Epidural analgesia (i.e., the provision of pain relief by continuous administration of pharmacological agents into the epidural space via an indwelling catheter) has become a widely used technique for the management of acute pain after surgery and trauma. Regardless of the analgesic agent used, location of catheter, or the type of surgery, it provides better pain relief than parenteral opioid administration.

Improved pain relief with epidural local anesthetics leads to a decreased incidence of pulmonary infection and other pulmonary complications overall when compared with systemic opioids. The combination of a low concentration of local anesthetic and opioid is superior to either of the drugs alone. The addition of small amounts of adrenaline (epinephrine) to such mixtures improves analgesia and reduces systemic opioid consumption. Administration of a local anesthetic into the thoracic epidural space results in improved bowel recovery, but this benefit is not consistent with lumbar administration. Adverse effects are uncommon but include permanent neurological damage, which is reported at 0.05–0.0005%, and epidural hematoma (0.0005%). Others include respiratory depression (1–15%) and hypotension (5–10%).

Systemic Analgesia

Necessary prerequisites for patient-orientated systemic pain therapy are good knowledge and understanding of the cause of pain (inflammation, spasm, type of operation or operative access, anxiety, or depression of the patient), the anatomy and pain transduction, and, based on this information, the necessary surgical, physical, psychological, or medical therapy. Whereas chronic pain treatment starts with nonpharmacological techniques (psychotherapy, TENS, etc.) followed by mild non-opioid analgesics, and, subsequently, strong opioids, the treatment of acute pain follows the reverse order (Fig. 7.3).

Strong opioids combined with NSAIDs are used as first-line therapy to control pain when intensity is highest. Analgesic drugs given by the intravenous route have a more rapid onset of action compared with most other routes of administration. Titration of opioid therapy for severe acute pain is best achieved using intermittent intravenous bolus doses (2–3 mg of morphine at 5 min intervals until relief of pain). Relative or absolute overdosing (also rapid injection) may lead to complications and side effects independent of the opioid used. However, the risk of overdosing with resultant respiratory

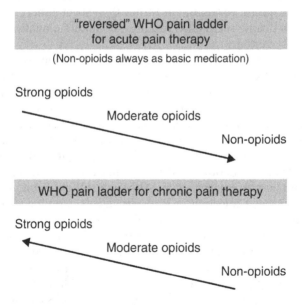

FIGURE 7.3. WHO's pain ladder of acute and chronic pain therapy.

depression is not an issue as long as the patient continues to experience pain. If it occurs, sufficient antagonists (naloxone 0.4 mg) should always be available and the sedation level should be assessed in parallel. Continuous infusion of opioids in the general ward setting is not recommended because of the increased risk of respiratory depression compared with other methods of parenteral opioid administration.

Non-opioid analgesics have an antipyretic and anti-inflammatory effect. They should be administered either solely (such as after minor operations) or in combination with opioids. Opioid and nonopioid drugs can be administered systemically by a number of different routes. The choice of route is determined by various factors including the overall condition of the patient but also by the ease of use, accessibility, speed of analgesic onset, duration of action, and patient acceptability. In general, the principle of individualization of dose and dosing intervals should apply to the administration of all analgesic drugs, whatever the route. Frequent assessment of the patient's pain and their response to treatment rather than strict adherence to a given dosing regimen is required if adequate analgesia is to be obtained.

Oral administration is straightforward, noninvasive, has good efficacy in most settings, and has a high patient acceptability. Other than in the treatment of severe acute pain, it is the route of choice for most analgesic drugs provided that there is no contraindication to its use. After major operations or trauma, the aim should be to change to the oral route as quickly as possible. The analgesic efficacy varies from one pain model to another and the administration of analgesics should be procedure specific. Although still used commonly, intramuscular injection of analgesic agents is no longer recommended because of the significant risk of abscess formation, nerve lesions, and necrosis. Subcutaneous injection shares the same problem as intramuscular administration that absorption may be impaired in situations of poor perfusion. This leads to inadequate early analgesia and late absorption of the drug depot when perfusion is re-established. Rectal administration of drugs is useful when other routes are unavailable. Transdermal routes for opioid administration (fentanyl or buprenorphine patches) are not recommended for acute pain management due to safety concerns (respiratory depression) and the difficulties in short-term dose adjustments that may be required for titration.

The general rule is that the patient should determine their analgesic requirement within given limitations for all routes of administration. Patient-controlled analgesia (PCA) refers to methods of pain relief that allow the patient to self-administer small doses of an analgesic agent as required. This is not necessarily associated only to the use of programmable infusion pumps. Adequate analgesia needs to be obtained prior to commencement of PCA. Initial instructions for bolus doses should take into account individual patient factors such as history of prior opioid use and patient age. Individual prescriptions may need to be adjusted and drug concentrations should be standardized within each institution to reduce programming errors. A background infusion is not recommended in acute pain management.

Organization of Acute Pain Management

Pain management is an interdisciplinary undertaking. Successful management of acute pain requires close liaison with all personnel involved in the care of the patient and should include surgeons, anesthesiologists, and nurses. Effective acute pain management will only result from appropriate education and organizational structures for the delivery of pain relief. Clear-cut responsibilities between disciplines are mandatory and this may differ between countries or even hospitals. Effective organizational structures for the delivery of pain relief are often more important than the analgesic techniques themselves. In some institutions, acute pain services (APS) are responsible for managing more advanced methods of pain relief such as PCA and epidural analgesia. There is a wide diversity of APS structures (from low-cost nurse-based through to multidisciplinary services) with different responsibilities. A recent review of publications analyzing the effectiveness of APS concluded that its implementation is associated with a significant improvement of pain relief with a possible reduction of postoperative nausea and vomiting.

Marked improvements in conventional methods of pain relief can be expected by the introduction of evidence-based clinical practice guidelines. However, it is the implementation of guidelines and not their development, which remains the greatest obstacle to their use. Professional bodies in a number of countries have published guidelines for the management of acute pain. A procedure-specific approach is highly recommended such as the online PROSPECT group (http://www.postoppain.org.htm). Resource availability, staff with pain management expertise, and the existence of formal quality assurance programs to monitor pain management are positive predictors of compliance with guidelines. Official guidelines need to be adapted for individual hospital requirements and the ward nurses play the most significant role in local adaptation. With their support, and that of clinical management and directors of surgical departments, national guidelines on acute pain management have been successfully translated into the initiative "Pain Free Clinic." The Cologne City Hospital, Merheim was the first in Germany to receive board certification by an external organization. This initiative can serve as a role model for other hospitals in improving the organization of acute pain management with benefit to the patients and the hospital.

Selected Readings

American Society of Anesthesiologists (2004) Practice guidelines for acute pain management in the perioperative setting. An updated report by the American Society of Anesthesiologists Task Force on Acute Pain Management. Anesthesiology 100:1573–1581

Australian and New Zealand College of Anaesthetists and Faculty of Pain Medicine (2005) Acute pain management: scientific evidence, 2nd edn. National Health and Medical Research Council. http://www.nhmrc.gov.au/publications/subjects/clinical.htm

Ballantyne IS, Carr DB, de Ferranti S, et al. (1998) The comparative effects of postoperative analgesic therapies on pulmonary outcome: cumulative meta-analyses of randomized, controlled trials. Anaesth Analg 86:598–612

Kehlet H (1997) Multimodal approaches to control postoperative pathophysiology and rehabilitation. Br J Anaesth 78:606–617

Kehlet H, Gray AW, Bonnett F, et al. (2005) A procedure specific systematic review and consensus recommendations for postoperative analgesia following laparoscopic cholecystectomy. Surg Endosc 19:1396–1415

Neugebauer E (2005) Initiative Schmerzfreie Klinik –(k)eine vision. Der Schmerz 19:557

Neugebauer E, Hempl K, Sauuerland ST, et al. (1998) Situation der perioperativen Schmerztherapie in Deutschland –Ergebnisse einer repra"sentativen, anonymen Umfrage von 1000 chirurgischen. Kliniken Chirurg 69:461–466

Veterans Health Administration D. o. D. Clinical practice guideline for management of postoperative pain (2002) http://www.oqp.med.va.gov/cqg/PAIN/PAIN_base.htm

Werner MU, Søholm L, Rotbøll-Nielssen, et al. (2002) Does an acute pain service improve postoperative outcome. Anaesth Analg 95:1361–1372

Zhao SZ, Chung F, Hanna P, et al. (2004) Dose-response relationship between opioids use and adverse effects after ambulatory surgery. Pain Symptom Manage 28:35–46

Index

Index